Understanding Cancer

Background, Clinical Trials, Research, and Prevention

snova
New York

Cancer Etiology, Diagnosis and Treatments Series

Pathways to Healing: Advancements in Cancer Therapy
Pranav Kumar Prabhakar, PhD
ISBN: 979-8-89530-735-9
eBook ISBN: 979-8-89530-828-8

Polymeric Nanocarriers in Cancer Treatment
Vijay Mishra, PhD and Yachana Mishra, PhD
ISBN: 979-8-89530-597-3
eBook ISBN: 979-8-89530-740-3

Nature's Arsenal Against Cancer: Harnessing the Power of Natural Compounds for Treatment and Prevention
Kumar Guarve, PhD, Ajmer Singh Grewal, PhD, Geeta Deswal, PhD and Ashwani K. Dhingra, PhD
ISBN: 979-8-89530-202-6
eBook ISBN: 979-8-89530-227-9

Current Trends in Breast Disease Management
Adem Aslan, Nazan Yurtcu, MD and Mustafa Can Güler
ISBN: 979-8-89113-875-9
eBook ISBN: 979-8-89113-949-7

More information about this series can be found at
https://novapublishers.com/product-category/series/cancer-etiology-diagnosis-and-treatments/

Angela C. Ray
Editor

Understanding Cancer

Background, Clinical Trials, Research, and Prevention

snova
New York

Library of Congress Cataloging-in-Publication Data

ISBN: 979-8-89530-769-4 (Hardcover)
ISBN: 979-8-89530-950-6 (eBook)

Published by Nova Science Publishers, Inc. † New York

Contents

Preface

Cancer is not a single disease, but rather a collection of related diseases that can occur almost anywhere in the body. At its core, cancer arises from changes in the genes that regulate how our body's cells function. Genes control how cells work; however, alterations in these genes can lead to cells malfunctioning—causing them to grow and divide uncontrollably or avoid programmed cell death. These abnormal cells can become cancerous. Understanding how genetic changes contribute to cancer is one way to grasp the disease, while analyzing cancer statistics provides another perspective. Symptoms and treatments vary depending on the type and stage of cancer. Common approaches include surgery, radiation, and chemotherapy, while some treatment plans may also involve hormone therapy, immunotherapy, biologic therapy, or stem cell transplantation.

Chapter 1

What Is Cancer?*

National Cancer Institute

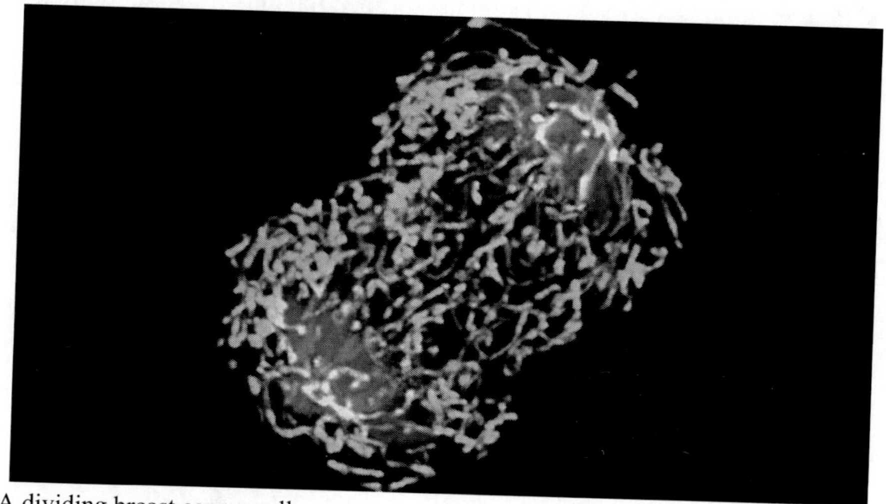

A dividing breast cancer cell.
Credit: National Cancer Institute / Univ. of Pittsburgh Cancer Institute.

The Definition of Cancer

Cancer is a disease in which some of the body's cells grow uncontrollably and spread to other parts of the body.

Cancer can start almost anywhere in the human body, which is made up of trillions of cells. Normally, human cells grow and multiply (through a

---

* This is an edited, reformatted and augmented version of National Cancer Institute Publication.

In: Understanding Cancer
Editor: Angela C. Ray
ISBN: 979-8-89530-769-4

process called cell division) to form new cells as the body needs them. When cells grow old or become damaged, they die, and new cells take their place.

Sometimes this orderly process breaks down, and abnormal or damaged cells grow and multiply when they shouldn't. These cells may form tumors, which are lumps of tissue. Tumors can be cancerous or not cancerous (benign).

Cancerous tumors spread into, or invade, nearby tissues and can travel to distant places in the body to form new tumors (a process called metastasis). Cancerous tumors may also be called malignant tumors. Many cancers form solid tumors, but cancers of the blood, such as leukemias, generally do not.

Benign tumors do not spread into, or invade, nearby tissues. When removed, benign tumors usually don't grow back, whereas cancerous tumors sometimes do. Benign tumors can sometimes be quite large, however. Some can cause serious symptoms or be life threatening, such as benign tumors in the brain.

Differences Between Cancer Cells and Normal Cells

Cancer cells differ from normal cells in many ways. For instance, cancer cells:

- grow in the absence of signals telling them to grow. Normal cells only grow when they receive such signals.
- ignore signals that normally tell cells to stop dividing or to die (a process known as programmed cell death, or apoptosis).
- invade into nearby areas and spread to other areas of the body. Normal cells stop growing when they encounter other cells, and most normal cells do not move around the body.
- tell blood vessels to grow toward tumors. These blood vessels supply tumors with oxygen and nutrients and remove waste products from tumors.
- hide from the immune system. The immune system normally eliminates damaged or abnormal cells.
- trick the immune system into helping cancer cells stay alive and grow. For instance, some cancer cells convince immune cells to protect the tumor instead of attacking it.
- accumulate multiple changes in their chromosomes, such as duplications and deletions of chromosome parts. Some cancer cells have double the normal number of chromosomes.

- rely on different kinds of nutrients than normal cells. In addition, some cancer cells make energy from nutrients in a different way than most normal cells. This lets cancer cells grow more quickly.

Many times, cancer cells rely so heavily on these abnormal behaviors that they can't survive without them. Researchers have taken advantage of this fact, developing therapies that target the abnormal features of cancer cells. For example, some cancer therapies prevent blood vessels from growing toward tumors, essentially starving the tumor of needed nutrients.

How Does Cancer Develop?

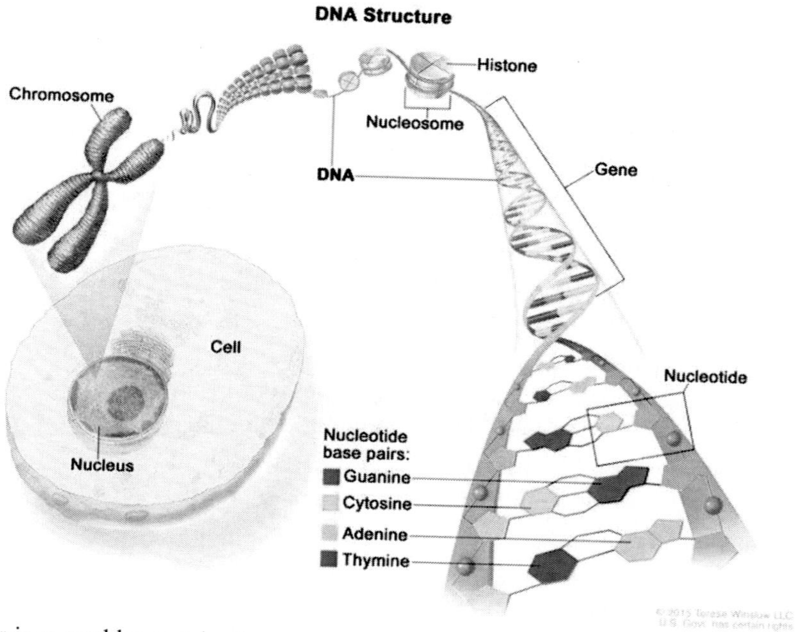

Cancer is caused by certain changes to genes, the basic physical units of inheritance. Genes are arranged in long strands of tightly packed DNA called chromosomes. Credit: © Terese Winslow

Cancer is a genetic disease—that is, it is caused by changes to genes that control the way our cells function, especially how they grow and divide.

Genetic changes that cause cancer can happen because:

- of errors that occur as cells divide.
- of damage to DNA caused by harmful substances in the environment, such as the chemicals in tobacco smoke and ultraviolet rays from the sun. (Our Cancer Causes and Prevention section has more information.)
- they were inherited from our parents.

The body normally eliminates cells with damaged DNA before they turn cancerous. But the body's ability to do so goes down as we age. This is part of the reason why there is a higher risk of cancer later in life.

Each person's cancer has a unique combination of genetic changes. As the cancer continues to grow, additional changes will occur. Even within the same tumor, different cells may have different genetic changes.

Fundamentals of Cancer

Types of Genes that Cause Cancer

The genetic changes that contribute to cancer tend to affect three main types of genes—proto-oncogenes, tumor suppressor genes, and DNA repair genes. These changes are sometimes called "drivers" of cancer.

Proto-oncogenes are involved in normal cell growth and division. However, when these genes are altered in certain ways or are more active than normal, they may become cancer-causing genes (or oncogenes), allowing cells to grow and survive when they should not.

Tumor suppressor genes are also involved in controlling cell growth and division. Cells with certain alterations in tumor suppressor genes may divide in an uncontrolled manner.

DNA repair genes are involved in fixing damaged DNA. Cells with mutations in these genes tend to develop additional mutations in other genes and changes in their chromosomes, such as duplications and deletions of chromosome parts. Together, these mutations may cause the cells to become cancerous.

As scientists have learned more about the molecular changes that lead to cancer, they have found that certain mutations commonly occur in many types of cancer. Now there are many cancer treatments available that target gene mutations found in cancer. A few of these treatments can be used by anyone with a cancer that has the targeted mutation, no matter where the cancer started growing.

When Cancer Spreads

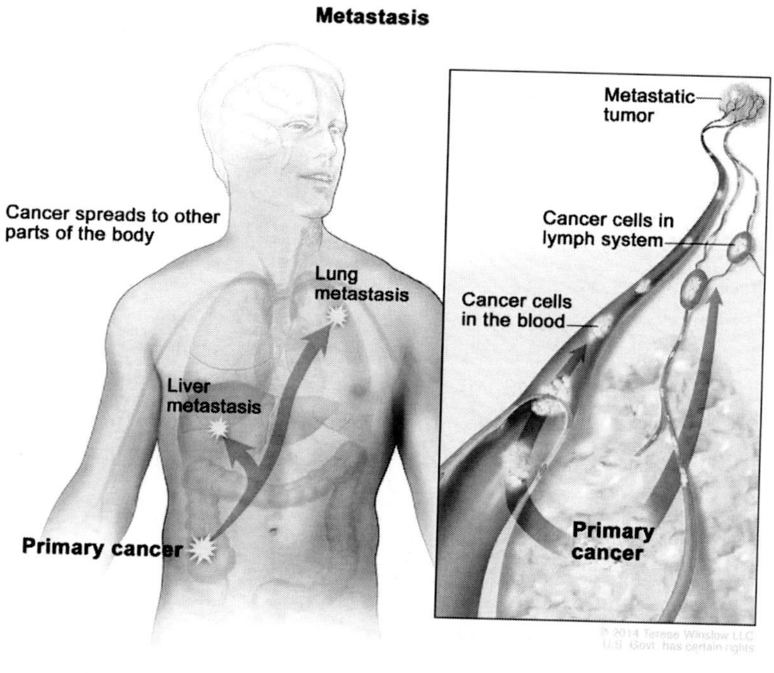

In metastasis, cancer cells break away from where they first formed and form new tumors in other parts of the body.
Credit: © Terese Winslow.

A cancer that has spread from the place where it first formed to another place in the body is called metastatic cancer. The process by which cancer cells spread to other parts of the body is called metastasis.

Metastatic cancer has the same name and the same type of cancer cells as the original, or primary, cancer. For example, breast cancer that forms a metastatic tumor in the lung is metastatic breast cancer, not lung cancer.

Under a microscope, metastatic cancer cells generally look the same as cells of the original cancer. Moreover, metastatic cancer cells and cells of the original cancer usually have some molecular features in common, such as the presence of specific chromosome changes.

In some cases, treatment may help prolong the lives of people with metastatic cancer. In other cases, the primary goal of treatment for metastatic cancer is to control the growth of the cancer or to relieve symptoms it is causing. Metastatic tumors can cause severe damage to how the body functions, and most people who die of cancer die of metastatic disease.

Tissue Changes that Are Not Cancer

Not every change in the body's tissues is cancer. Some tissue changes may develop into cancer if they are not treated, however. Here are some examples of tissue changes that are not cancer but, in some cases, are monitored because they could become cancer:

- *Hyperplasia* occurs when cells within a tissue multiply faster than normal and extra cells build up. However, the cells and the way the tissue is organized still look normal under a microscope. Hyperplasia can be caused by several factors or conditions, including chronic irritation.
- *Dysplasia* is a more advanced condition than hyperplasia. In dysplasia, there is also a buildup of extra cells. But the cells look abnormal and there are changes in how the tissue is organized. In general, the more abnormal the cells and tissue look, the greater the chance that cancer will form. Some types of dysplasia may need to be monitored or treated, but others do not. An example of dysplasia is an abnormal mole (called a dysplastic nevus) that forms on the skin. A dysplastic nevus can turn into melanoma, although most do not.
- *Carcinoma* in situ is an even more advanced condition. Although it is sometimes called stage 0 cancer, it is not cancer because the abnormal cells do not invade nearby tissue the way that cancer cells do. But because some carcinomas in situ may become cancer, they are usually treated.

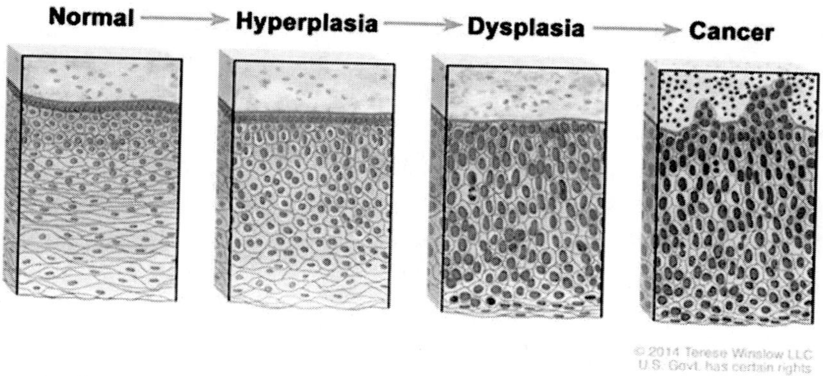

Normal cells may become cancer cells. Before cancer cells form in tissues of the body, the cells go through abnormal changes called hyperplasia and dysplasia. In hyperplasia, there is an increase in the number of cells in an organ or tissue that appear normal under a microscope. In dysplasia, the cells look abnormal under a microscope but are not cancer. Hyperplasia and dysplasia may or may not become cancer.
Credit: © Terese Winslow.

Types of Cancer

There are more than 100 types of cancer. Types of cancer are usually named for the organs or tissues where the cancers form. For example, lung cancer starts in the lung, and brain cancer starts in the brain. Cancers also may be described by the type of cell that formed them, such as an epithelial cell or a squamous cell.

You can search NCI's website for information on specific types of cancer based on the cancer's location in the body or by using our A to Z List of Cancers. We also have information on childhood cancers and cancers in adolescents and young adults.

Here are some categories of cancers that begin in specific types of cells:

Carcinoma

Carcinomas are the most common type of cancer. They are formed by epithelial cells, which are the cells that cover the inside and outside surfaces of the body. There are many types of epithelial cells, which often have a column-like shape when viewed under a microscope.

Carcinomas that begin in different epithelial cell types have specific names:

Adenocarcinoma is a cancer that forms in epithelial cells that produce fluids or mucus. Tissues with this type of epithelial cell are sometimes called glandular tissues. Most cancers of the breast, colon, and prostate are adenocarcinomas.

Basal cell carcinoma is a cancer that begins in the lower or basal (base) layer of the epidermis, which is a person's outer layer of skin.

Squamous cell carcinoma is a cancer that forms in squamous cells, which are epithelial cells that lie just beneath the outer surface of the skin. Squamous cells also line many other organs, including the stomach, intestines, lungs, bladder, and kidneys. Squamous cells look flat, like fish scales, when viewed under a microscope. Squamous cell carcinomas are sometimes called epidermoid carcinomas.

Transitional cell carcinoma is a cancer that forms in a type of epithelial tissue called transitional epithelium, or urothelium. This tissue, which is made up of many layers of epithelial cells that can get bigger and smaller, is found in the linings of the bladder, ureters, and part of the kidneys (renal pelvis), and a few other organs. Some cancers of the bladder, ureters, and kidneys are transitional cell carcinomas.

Sarcoma

Sarcomas are cancers that form in bone and soft tissues, including muscle, fat, blood vessels, lymph vessels, and fibrous tissue (such as tendons and ligaments).

Osteosarcoma is the most common cancer of bone. The most common types of soft tissue sarcoma are leiomyosarcoma, Kaposi sarcoma, malignant fibrous histiocytoma, liposarcoma, and dermatofibrosarcoma protuberans.

Our page on soft tissue sarcoma has more information.

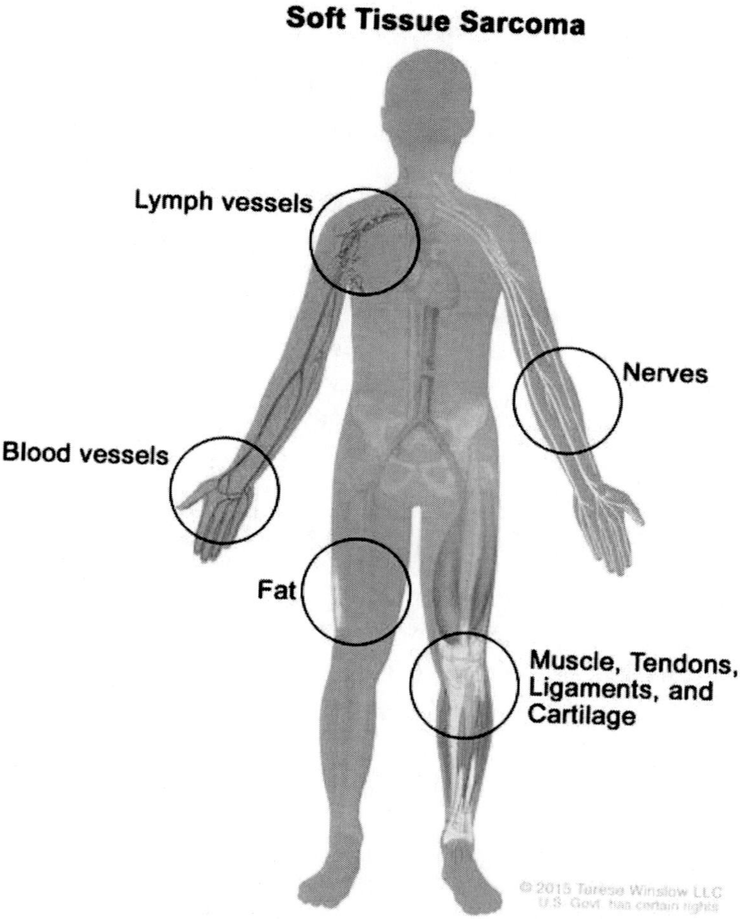

Soft tissue sarcoma forms in soft tissues of the body, including muscle, tendons, fat, blood vessels, lymph vessels, nerves, and tissue around joints.
Credit: © Terese Winslow.

Leukemia

Cancers that begin in the blood-forming tissue of the bone marrow are called leukemias. These cancers do not form solid tumors. Instead, large numbers of abnormal white blood cells (leukemia cells and leukemic blast cells) build up in the blood and bone marrow, crowding out normal blood cells. The low level of normal blood cells can make it harder for the body to get oxygen to its tissues, control bleeding, or fight infections.

There are four common types of leukemia, which are grouped based on how quickly the disease gets worse (acute or chronic) and on the type of blood cell the cancer starts in (lymphoblastic or myeloid). Acute forms of leukemia grow quickly and chronic forms grow more slowly.

Our page on leukemia has more information.

Lymphoma

Lymphoma is cancer that begins in lymphocytes (T cells or B cells). These are disease-fighting white blood cells that are part of the immune system. In lymphoma, abnormal lymphocytes build up in lymph nodes and lymph vessels, as well as in other organs of the body.

There are two main types of lymphoma:

Hodgkin lymphoma – People with this disease have abnormal lymphocytes that are called Reed-Sternberg cells. These cells usually form from B cells.

Non-Hodgkin lymphoma – This is a large group of cancers that start in lymphocytes. The cancers can grow quickly or slowly and can form from B cells or T cells.

Our page on lymphoma has more information.

Multiple Myeloma

Multiple myeloma is cancer that begins in plasma cells, another type of immune cell. The abnormal plasma cells, called myeloma cells, build up in the bone marrow and form tumors in bones all through the body. Multiple myeloma is also called plasma cell myeloma and Kahler disease.

Our page on multiple myeloma and other plasma cell neoplasms has more information.

Melanoma

Melanoma is cancer that begins in cells that become melanocytes, which are specialized cells that make melanin (the pigment that gives skin its color). Most melanomas form on the skin, but melanomas can also form in other pigmented tissues, such as the eye.

Our pages on skin cancer and intraocular melanoma have more information.

Brain and Spinal Cord Tumors

There are different types of brain and spinal cord tumors. These tumors are named based on the type of cell in which they formed and where the tumor first formed in the central nervous system. For example, an astrocytic tumor begins in star-shaped brain cells called astrocytes, which help keep nerve cells healthy. Brain tumors can be benign (not cancer) or malignant (cancer).

Our page on brain and spinal cord tumors has more information.

Other Types of Tumors

Germ Cell Tumors

Germ cell tumors are a type of tumor that begins in the cells that give rise to sperm or eggs. These tumors can occur almost anywhere in the body and can be either benign or malignant.

Our page of cancers by body location/system includes a list of germ cell tumors with links to more information.

Neuroendocrine Tumors

Neuroendocrine tumors form from cells that release hormones into the blood in response to a signal from the nervous system. These tumors, which may make higher-than-normal amounts of hormones, can cause many different symptoms. Neuroendocrine tumors may be benign or malignant.

Our definition of neuroendocrine tumors has more information.

Carcinoid Tumors

Carcinoid tumors are a type of neuroendocrine tumor. They are slow-growing tumors that are usually found in the gastrointestinal system (most often in the rectum and small intestine). Carcinoid tumors may spread to the liver or other sites in the body, and they may secrete substances such as serotonin or prostaglandins, causing carcinoid syndrome.

Our page on gastrointestinal neuroendocrine tumors has more information.

Chapter 2

Causes and Prevention*

National Cancer Institute

Cancer prevention is action taken to lower the risk of getting cancer. This can include maintaining a healthy lifestyle, avoiding exposure to known cancer-causing substances, and taking medicines or vaccines that can prevent cancer from developing.

Risk Factors for Cancer

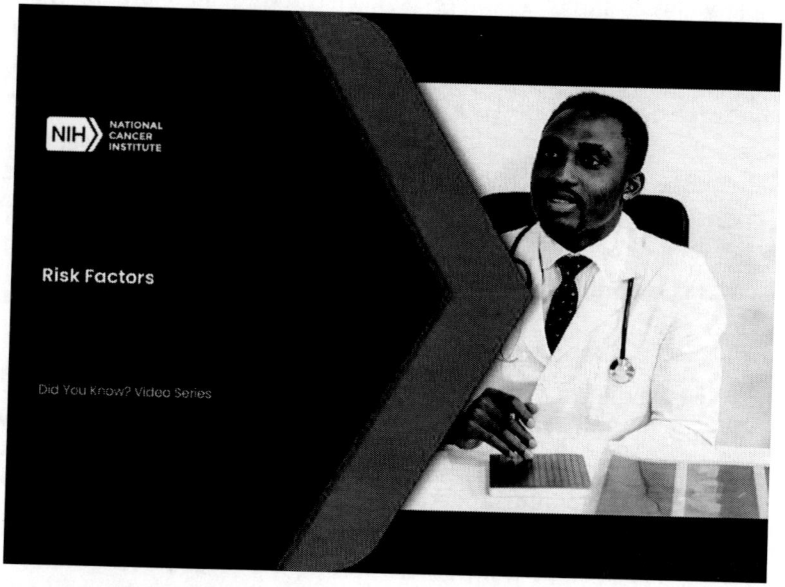

* This is an edited, reformatted and augmented version of National Cancer Institute Publication.

In: Understanding Cancer
Editor: Angela C. Ray
ISBN: 979-8-89530-769-4

Risk Factors for Cancer | Did You Know?

Aspects of a person's age, family history, lifestyle, and environment can increase the risk of developing cancer. Learn more from this Did You Know? video produced by NCI's Surveillance, Epidemiology, and End Results (SEER) program.

It is usually not possible to know exactly why one person develops cancer and another doesn't. But research has shown that certain risk factors may increase a person's chances of developing cancer. (There are also factors that are linked to a lower risk of cancer. These are sometimes called protective risk factors, or just protective factors.)

Cancer risk factors include exposure to chemicals or other substances, as well as certain behaviors. They also include things people cannot control, like age and family history. A family history of certain cancers can be a sign of a possible inherited cancer syndrome. (See the Hereditary Cancer Syndromes section for more information about inherited genetic mutations that can cause cancer.)

Most cancer risk (and protective) factors are initially identified in epidemiology studies. In these studies, scientists look at large groups of people and compare those who develop cancer with those who don't. These studies may show that the people who develop cancer are more or less likely to behave in certain ways or to be exposed to certain substances than those who do not develop cancer.

Such studies, on their own, cannot prove that a behavior or substance causes cancer. For example, the finding could be a result of chance, or the true risk factor could be something other than the suspected risk factor. But findings of this type sometimes get attention in the media, and this can lead to wrong ideas about how cancer starts and spreads. (See the Common Cancer Myths and Misconceptions page for more information.)

When many studies all point to a similar association between a potential risk factor and an increased risk of cancer, and when a possible mechanism exists that could explain how the risk factor could actually cause cancer, scientists can be more confident about the relationship between the two.

The list below includes the most-studied known or suspected risk factors for cancer. Although some of these risk factors can be avoided, others—such as growing older—cannot. Limiting your exposure to avoidable risk factors may lower your risk of developing certain cancers.

- Age
- Alcohol

- Cancer-Causing Substances
- Chronic Inflammation
- Diet
- Hormones
- Immunosuppression
- Infectious Agents
- Obesity
- Radiation
- Sunlight
- Tobacco

The Genetics of Cancer

- Is cancer a genetic disease?
- Is cancer hereditary?
- What is a family cancer syndrome?
- Should I get genetic testing for cancer risk?
- How can I find out what genetic changes are in my cancer?
- Who can see my genetic test results?
- How do genetic changes cause cancer?
- What kinds of genetic changes cause cancer?

Is Cancer a Genetic Disease?

Yes, cancer is a genetic disease. It is caused by changes in genes that control the way cells grow and multiply. Cells are the building blocks of your body. Each cell has a copy of your genes, which act like an instruction manual.

Genes are sections of DNA that carry instructions to make a protein or several proteins. Scientists have found hundreds of DNA and genetic changes (also called variants, mutations, or alterations) that help cancer form, grow, and spread.

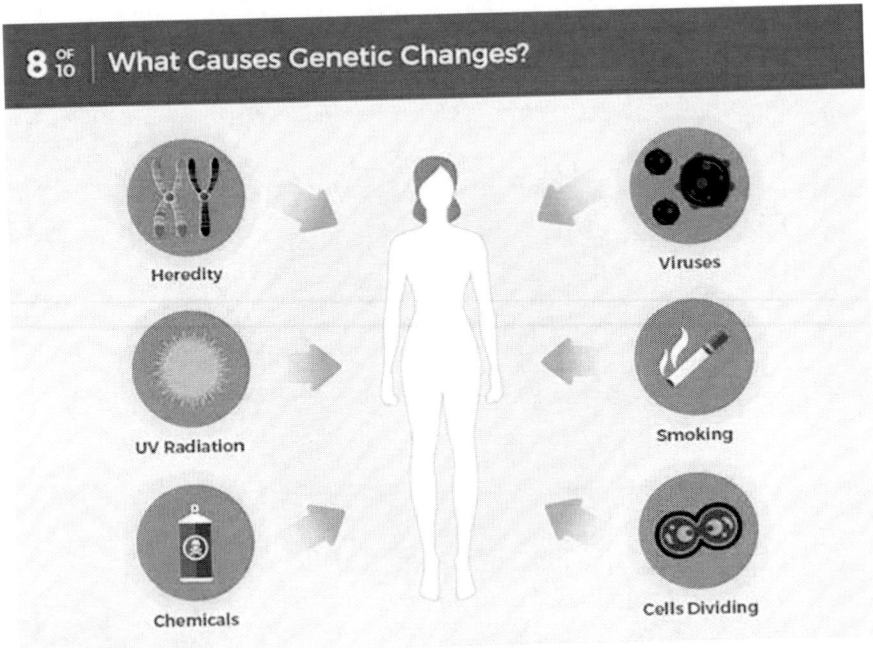

Genetic changes that cause cancer can be inherited or arise from certain environmental exposures. Genetic changes can also happen because of errors that occur as cells divide.
Credit: National Cancer Institute.

Cancer-related genetic changes can occur because:

- random mistakes in our DNA happen as our cells multiply
- our DNA is altered by carcinogens in our environment, such as chemicals in tobacco smoke, UV rays from the sun, and the human papillomavirus (HPV)
- they were inherited from one of our parents

DNA changes, whether caused by a random mistake or by a carcinogen, can happen throughout our lives and even in the womb. While most genetic changes aren't harmful on their own, an accumulation of genetic changes over many years can turn healthy cells into cancerous cells. The vast majority of cancers occur by chance as a result of this process over time.

Is Cancer Hereditary?

Cancer itself can't be passed down from parents to children. And genetic changes in tumor cells can't be passed down. But a genetic change that increases the risk of cancer can be passed down (inherited) if it is present in a parent's egg or sperm cells.

For example, if a parent passes a mutated BRCA1 or BRCA2 gene to their child, the child will have a much higher risk of developing breast and several other cancers.

That's why cancer sometimes appears to run in families. Up to 10% of all cancers may be caused by inherited genetic changes.

Inheriting a cancer-related genetic change doesn't mean you will definitely get cancer. It means that your risk of getting cancer is increased.

What Is a Family Cancer Syndrome?

A family cancer syndrome, also called a hereditary cancer syndrome, is a rare disorder in which family members have a higher-than-average risk of developing a certain type or types of cancer. Family cancer syndromes are caused by inherited genetic variants in certain cancer-related genes.

With some family cancer syndromes, people tend to develop cancer at an early age or have other noncancer health conditions.

For example, familial adenomatous polyposis (FAP) is a family cancer syndrome caused by certain inherited changes in the *APC* gene. People with FAP have a very high chance of developing colorectal cancer at an early age and are also at risk of developing other kinds of cancer.

But not all cancers that appear to "run in families" are caused by family cancer syndromes. A shared environment or habits, such as exposure to air pollution or tobacco use, may cause the same kind of cancer to develop among family members.

Also, multiple family members may develop common cancers, such as prostate cancer, just by chance. Cancer can also run in a family if family members have a combination of many genetic variants that each have a very small cancer risk.

Should I Get Genetic Testing for Cancer Risk?

Certain genetic tests can show if you've inherited a genetic change that increases your risk of cancer. This testing is usually done with a small sample of blood, but it can sometimes be done with saliva, cells from inside the cheek, or skin cells.

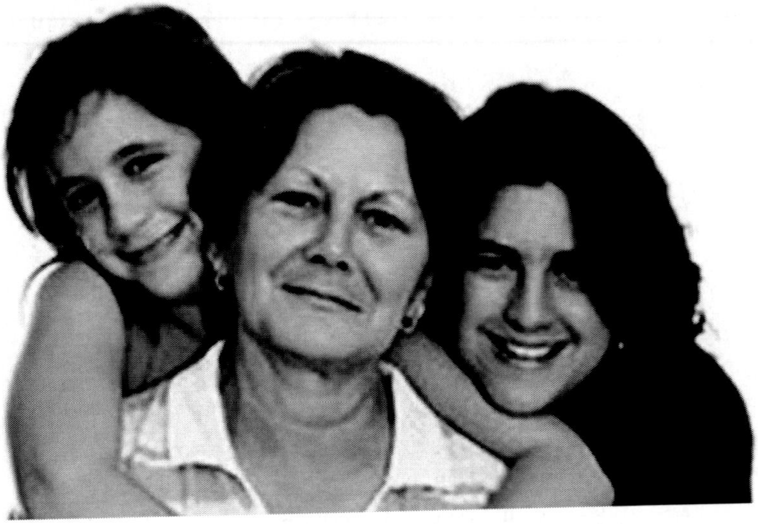

Genetic tests can help families with a history of breast and ovarian cancer make screening and treatment decisions.

Not everyone needs to get genetic testing for cancer risk. Your doctor or health care provider can help you decide if you should get tested for genetic changes that increase cancer risk. They will likely ask if you have certain patterns in your personal or family medical history, such as cancer at an unusually young age or several relatives with the same kind of cancer.

If your doctor recommends genetic testing, talking with a genetic counselor can help you consider the potential risks, benefits, and drawbacks of genetic testing in your situation. After testing, a genetic counselor, doctor, or other health care professional trained in genetics can help you understand what the test results mean for you and for your family members.

Although it's possible to order an at-home genetic test on your own, these tests have many drawbacks and are *not* generally recommended as a way to see whether you have inherited a genetic change that increases cancer risk.

For more information on what tests are available and who may want to consider them, see Genetic Testing for Inherited Cancer Risk.

How Can I Find Out What Genetic Changes Are in My Cancer?

If you have cancer, a different type of genetic test called a biomarker test can identify genetic changes that may be driving the growth of your cancer. This information can help your doctors decide which therapy might work best for you or if you may be able to enroll in a particular clinical trial. For more information, see Biomarker Testing for Cancer Treatment. Biomarker testing may also be called tumor profiling or molecular profiling.

Biomarker testing is different from the genetic testing that is used to find out if you have an inherited genetic change that makes you more likely to get cancer. Biomarker testing is done using a sample of your cancer cells—either a small piece of a tumor or a sample of your blood.

In some cases, the results of a biomarker test might suggest that you have an inherited mutation that increases cancer risk. If that happens, you may need to get another genetic test to confirm whether you truly have an inherited mutation that increases cancer risk.

Who Can See My Genetic Test Results?

Your genetic counselor, doctors, and other health care professionals might see your genetic test results. In addition, your health insurance company has legitimate, legal access to your medical records.

Legal protections prevent discrimination on the basis of genetic test results, including the *Genetic Information Nondiscrimination Act of 2008 (GINA) and the Privacy Rule of the Health Information Portability and Accountability Act of 1996 (HIPAA).*

How Do Genetic Changes Cause Cancer?

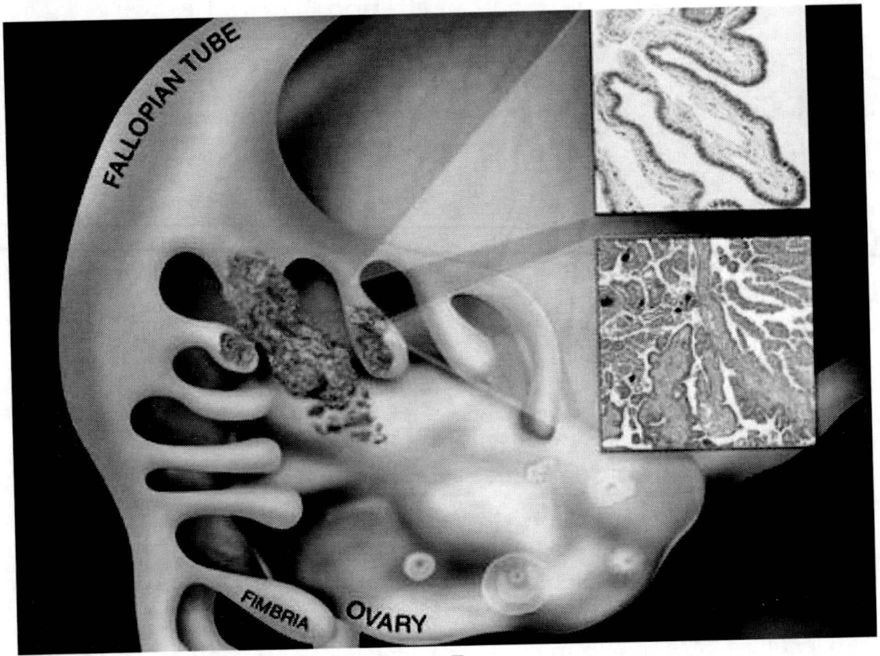

Study Helps Explain How Ovarian Cancer Forms.
The findings could potentially help doctors detect the cancer earlier.

Genetic changes can lead to cancer if they alter the way your cells grow and spread. Most cancer-causing DNA changes occur in genes, which are sections of DNA that carry the instructions to make proteins or specialized RNA such as microRNA.

For example, some DNA changes raise the levels of proteins that tell cells to keep growing. Other DNA changes lower the levels of proteins that tell cells when to stop growing. And some DNA changes stop proteins that tell cells to self-destruct when they are damaged.

For a healthy cell to turn cancerous, scientists think that more than one DNA change has to occur. People who have inherited a cancer-related genetic change need fewer additional changes to develop cancer. However, they may never develop these changes or get cancer.

As cancer cells divide, they acquire more DNA changes over time. Two cancer cells in the same tumor can have different DNA changes. In addition, every person with cancer has a unique combination of DNA changes in their cancer.

For more information on the biological changes that make cells cancerous, see What is Cancer? Differences between Cancer Cells and Normal Cells.

What Kinds of Genetic Changes Cause Cancer?

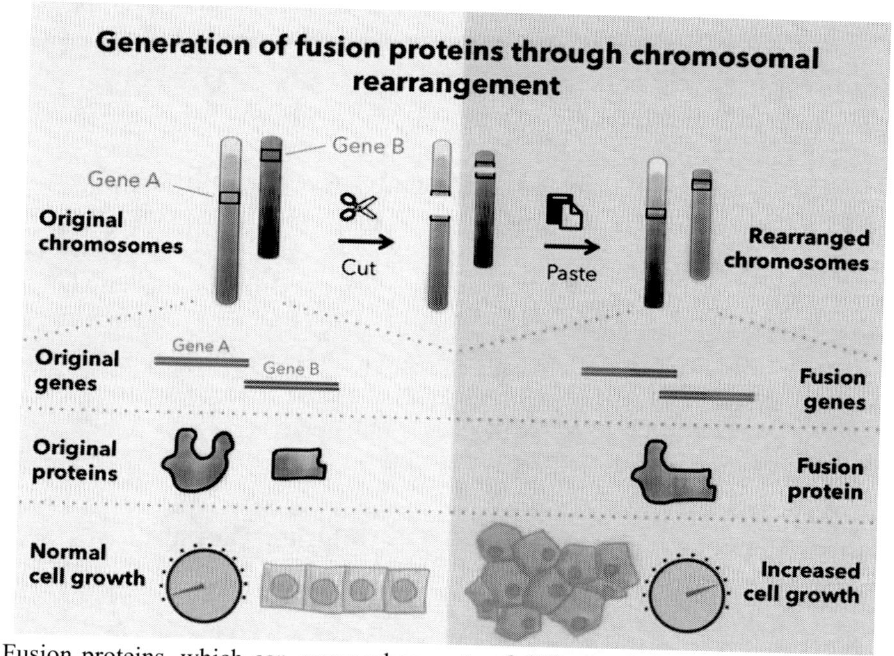

Fusion proteins, which can occur when parts of different chromosomal regions are joined, may drive the development of many cancers in children.

Credit: Shannon McArdel, Ph.D. Harvard University SITN Blog, June 2017. CC BY-NC-SA 4.0.

Multiple kinds of genetic changes can lead to cancer. One genetic change, called a DNA mutation or genetic variant, is a change in the DNA code, like a typo in the sequence of DNA letters.

Some variants affect just one DNA letter, called a nucleotide. A nucleotide may be missing, or it may be replaced by another nucleotide. These are called point mutations.

For example, around 5% of people with cancer have a point mutation in the KRAS gene that replaces the DNA letter G with AExit Disclaimer. This single letter change creates an abnormal KRAS protein that constantly tells cells to grow.

Cancer-causing genetic changes can also occur when segments of DNA—sometimes very large ones—are rearranged, deleted, or copied. These are called chromosomal rearrangements.

For example, most chronic myelogenous leukemias (a type of blood cancer) are caused by a chromosomal rearrangement that places part of the *BCR* gene next to the *ABL* gene. This rearrangement creates an abnormal protein, called BCR-ABL, that makes leukemia cells grow out of control.

Some cancer-causing DNA changes occur outside genes, in sections of DNA that act like "on" or "off" switches for nearby genes. For example, some brain cancer cells have multiple copies of "on" switches next to genes that drive cell growth.

Other DNA changes, known as epigenetic changes, can also cause cancer. Unlike genetic variants, epigenetic changes (sometimes called epimutations) may be reversible and they don't affect the DNA code. Instead, epigenetic changes affect how DNA is packed into the nucleus. By changing how DNA is packaged, epigenetic changes can alter how much protein a gene makes.

Some substances and chemicals in the environment that cause genetic changes can also cause epigenetic changes, such as tobacco smoke, heavy metals like cadmium, and viruses like Epstein-Barr virus.

Cancer Prevention Overview (PDQ®)–Patient Version

- Go to Health Professional Version
- What Is Prevention?
- Carcinogenesis
- Risk Factors
- Interventions That Are Known to Lower Cancer Risk
- Interventions That Are Not Known to Lower Cancer Risk
- About This PDQ Summary

What Is Prevention?

Cancer prevention is action taken to lower the chance of getting cancer. In 2023, about 1.9 million people will be diagnosed with cancer in the United States. In addition to the physical problems and emotional distress caused by cancer, the high costs of care are also a burden to patients, their families, and to the public. By preventing cancer, the number of new cases of cancer is lowered. Hopefully, this will reduce the burden of cancer and lower the number of deaths caused by cancer.

Cancer is not a single disease but a group of related diseases. Many things in our genes, our lifestyle, and the environment around us may increase or decrease our risk of getting cancer.

Scientists are studying many different ways to help prevent cancer, including the following:

- Ways to avoid or control things known to cause cancer.
- Changes in diet and lifestyle.
- Finding precancerous conditions early. Precancerous conditions are conditions that may become cancer.
- Chemoprevention (medicines to treat a precancerous condition or to keep cancer from starting).
- Risk-reducing surgery.

Carcinogenesis

Key Points

- Carcinogenesis is the process in which normal cells turn into cancer cells.
- Changes (mutations) in genes occur during carcinogenesis.

Carcinogenesis Is the Process in Which Normal Cells Turn into Cancer Cells

Carcinogenesis is the series of steps that take place as a normal cell becomes a cancer cell. Cells are the smallest units of the body and they make up the body's tissues. Each cell contains genes that guide the way the body grows, develops, and repairs itself. There are many genes that control whether a cell lives or dies, divides (multiplies), or takes on special functions, such as becoming a nerve cell or a muscle cell.

Changes (Mutations) in Genes Occur During Carcinogenesis

Changes (mutations) in genes can cause normal controls in cells to break down. When this happens, cells do not die when they should and new cells are produced when the body does not need them. The buildup of extra cells may cause a mass (tumor) to form.

Tumors can be benign or malignant (cancerous). Malignant tumor cells invade nearby tissues and spread to other parts of the body. Benign tumor cells do not invade nearby tissues or spread.

Risk Factors

Key Points

- Factors that are known to increase the risk of cancer
    - Cigarette smoking and tobacco use
    - Infections
    - Radiation
    - Immunosuppressive medicines after organ transplant
- Factors that may affect the risk of cancer
    - Diet
    - Alcohol
    - Physical activity
    - Obesity
    - Diabetes
    - Environmental risk factors

Scientists study risk factors and protective factors to find ways to prevent new cancers from starting. Anything that increases your chance of developing cancer is called a cancer risk factor; anything that decreases your chance of developing cancer is called a cancer protective factor.

Some risk factors for cancer can be avoided, but many cannot. For example, both smoking and inheriting certain genes are risk factors for some types of cancer, but only smoking can be avoided. Risk factors that a person can control are called modifiable risk factors.

Many other factors in our environment, diet, and lifestyle may cause or prevent cancer. This summary reviews only the major cancer risk factors and protective factors that can be controlled or changed to reduce the risk of cancer. Risk factors that are not described in the summary include certain sexual behaviors, the use of estrogen, and being exposed to certain substances at work or to certain chemicals.

Factors That Are Known to Increase the Risk of Cancer

Cigarette Smoking and Tobacco Use

Tobacco use is strongly linked to an increased risk for many kinds of cancer. Smoking cigarettes is the leading cause of the following types of cancer:

- Acute myelogenous leukemia (AML).
- Bladder cancer.
- Cervical cancer.
- Esophageal cancer.
- Kidney cancer.
- Lung cancer.
- Oral cavity cancer.
- Pancreatic cancer.
- Stomach cancer.

Not smoking or quitting smoking lowers the risk of getting cancer and dying from cancer. Scientists believe that cigarette smoking causes about 30% of all cancer deaths in the United States.

See the following PDQ summaries for more information:

- Lung Cancer Prevention
- Lung Cancer Screening
- Cigarette Smoking: Health Risks and How to Quit

Infections

Certain viruses and bacteria are able to cause cancer. Examples of cancer-causing viruses and bacteria include:

- Human papillomavirus (HPV) increases the risk for cancers of the cervix, penis, vagina, anus, and oropharynx.
- Hepatitis B and hepatitis C viruses increase the risk for liver cancer.
- Epstein-Barr virus increases the risk for Burkitt lymphoma.
- Helicobacter pylori increases the risk for gastric cancer.

Two vaccines to prevent infection by cancer-causing agents have been developed and approved by the US Food and Drug Administration (FDA). One is a vaccine to prevent infection with hepatitis B virus. The other protects against infection with strains of human papillomavirus (HPV) that cause cervical cancer. Scientists continue to work on vaccines against infections that cause cancer.

See the following PDQ summaries for more information:

- Cervical Cancer Causes, Risk Factors, and Prevention
- Cervical Cancer Screening
- Liver Cancer Causes, Risk Factors, and Prevention
- Stomach Cancer Causes and Risk Factors
- Oral Cavity, Oropharyngeal, Hypopharyngeal, and Laryngeal Cancers Prevention

Radiation

Being exposed to radiation is a known cause of cancer. There are two main types of radiation linked with an increased risk of cancer:

- Ultraviolet radiation from sunlight: This is the main cause of nonmelanoma skin cancers.
- Ionizing radiation including:
    - Medical radiation from tests to diagnose cancer such as x-rays, CT scans, fluoroscopy, and nuclear medicine scans.
    - Radon gas in our homes.

Scientists believe that ionizing radiation causes leukemia, thyroid cancer, and breast cancer in women. Ionizing radiation may also be linked to myeloma and cancers of the lung, stomach, colon, esophagus, bladder, and ovary. Being exposed to radiation from diagnostic x-rays increases the risk of cancer in patients and x-ray technicians. Diagnostic radiation in children and adolescents has been linked with a higher risk of cancers at a young age.

The growing use of CT scans over the last 20 years has increased exposure to ionizing radiation. The risk of cancer also increases with the number of CT scans a patient has and the radiation dose used each time.

See the following PDQ summaries for more information:

- Breast Cancer Prevention
- Breast Cancer Screening
- Skin Cancer Prevention
- Lung Cancer Prevention

Immunosuppressive Medicines After Organ Transplant

Immunosuppressive medicines are used after an organ has been transplanted from one person to another. These medicines stop an organ that has been transplanted from being rejected. These medicines decrease the body's immune response to help keep the organ from being rejected. Immunosuppressive medicines are linked to an increased risk of cancer because they lower the body's ability to keep cancer from forming. The risk of cancer, especially cancer caused by a virus, is higher in the first 6 months after organ transplant, but the risk lasts for many years.

Factors That May Affect the Risk of Cancer

Diet

The foods that you eat on a regular basis make up your diet. Diet is being studied as a risk factor for cancer. It is hard to study the effects of diet on cancer because a person's diet includes foods that may protect against cancer and foods that may increase the risk of cancer.

It is also hard for people who take part in the studies to keep track of what they eat over a long period of time. This may explain why studies have different results about how diet affects the risk of cancer.

Some studies have shown that a diet high in fat, proteins, calories, and red meat increases the risk of colorectal cancer, but other studies have not shown this.

It is not known if a diet low in fat and high in fiber, fruits, and vegetables lowers the risk of colorectal cancer.

Alcohol

Studies have shown that drinking alcohol is linked to an increased risk of the following types of cancers:

- Oral cancer.
- Esophageal cancer.
- Breast cancer.
- Colorectal cancer (in men).

Drinking alcohol may also increase the risk of liver cancer and female colorectal cancer.

See the following PDQ summaries for more information:

- Breast Cancer Prevention
- Colorectal Cancer Prevention
- Lung Cancer Prevention
- Esophageal Cancer Prevention
- Oral Cavity, Oropharyngeal, Hypopharyngeal, and Laryngeal Cancers Prevention
- Liver Cancer Causes, Risk Factors, and Prevention

Physical Activity

Studies show that people who are physically active have a lower risk of certain cancers than those who are not. It is not known if physical activity itself is the reason for this.

Some studies show that physical activity protects against postmenopausal breast cancer and endometrial cancer.

See the following PDQ summaries for more information:

- Breast Cancer Prevention
- Colorectal Cancer Prevention
- Endometrial Cancer Prevention

Obesity

Studies show that obesity is linked to a higher risk of the following types of cancer:

- Postmenopausal breast cancer.
- Colorectal cancer.
- Endometrial cancer.
- Esophageal cancer.
- Kidney cancer.
- Pancreatic cancer.

Some studies show that obesity is also a risk factor for cancer of the gallbladder and liver cancer.

Studies have shown that people who lose weight decrease their risk of these cancers.

See the following PDQ summaries for more information:

- Breast Cancer Prevention
- Colorectal Cancer Prevention
- Endometrial Cancer Prevention
- Lung Cancer Prevention

Diabetes

Some studies show that having diabetes may slightly increase the risk of having the following types of cancer:

- Bladder cancer.
- Breast cancer in women.
- Colorectal cancer.

- Endometrial cancer.
- Liver cancer.
- Lung cancer.
- Oral cancer.
- Oropharyngeal cancer.
- Ovarian cancer.
- Pancreatic cancer.

Diabetes and cancer share some of the same risk factors. These risk factors include the following:

- Being older.
- Having obesity.
- Smoking.
- Not eating a healthy diet.
- Not exercising.

Because diabetes and cancer share these risk factors, it is hard to know whether the risk of cancer is increased more by diabetes or by these risk factors.

Studies are being done to see how medicine that is used to treat diabetes affects cancer risk.

Environmental Risk Factors

Being exposed to chemicals and other substances in the environment has been linked to some cancers:

- Links between air pollution and cancer risk have been found. These include links between lung cancer and secondhand tobacco smoke, outdoor air pollution, and asbestos.
- Drinking water that contains a large amount of arsenic has been linked to skin, bladder, and lung cancers.

Studies have been done to see if pesticides and other pollutants increase the risk of cancer. The results of those studies have been unclear because other factors can change the results of the studies.

Interventions That Are Known to Lower Cancer Risk

Key Points

- Chemoprevention is being studied in people who have a high risk of developing cancer.
- Studies have shown that weight loss surgery lowers cancer risk.

An intervention is a treatment or action taken to prevent or treat disease, or improve health in other ways. Many studies are being done to find ways to keep cancer from starting or coming back.

Chemoprevention Is Being Studied in People Who Have a High Risk of Developing Cancer

Chemoprevention is the use of substances to lower the risk of cancer, or keep it from recurring. The substances may be natural or made in the laboratory. Some chemopreventive agents are tested in people who are at high risk for a certain type of cancer. The risk may be because of a precancerous condition, family history, or lifestyle factors.

Taking one of the following agents may lower the risk of cancer:

- Selective estrogen receptor modulators (SERMS) such as tamoxifen or raloxifene have been shown to reduce the risk of breast cancer in women at high risk. SERMS may cause side effects, such as hot flashes, so they are not often used for prevention of cancer. For more information, see Breast Cancer Prevention.
- Finasteride has been shown to lower the risk of prostate cancer. For more information, see Prostate Cancer Prevention.
- COX-2 inhibitors may prevent colon and breast cancer. COX-2 inhibitors may cause heart problems. Because COX-2 inhibitors may cause heart problems there have not been many studies on their use to prevent cancer. For more information, see Colorectal Cancer Prevention and Breast Cancer Prevention.

Studies Have Shown That Weight Loss Surgery Lowers Cancer Risk

Weight loss surgery, also called bariatric surgery, is a procedure that people with obesity can have to lose weight and improve their overall health and quality of life. The surgery changes the anatomy of the stomach or changes the way the body absorbs nutrients. A person who undergoes this procedure will lose a lot of weight and as a result, will have a decreased risk of cancers that are linked to being overweight.

See the NCI website for more information about cancer prevention.

Interventions That Are Not Known to Lower Cancer Risk

Key Points

- Aspirin has not been shown to prevent most cancers.
- Vitamin and dietary supplements have not been shown to prevent cancer.
- New ways to prevent cancer are being studied in clinical trials.

Aspirin Has Not Been Shown to Prevent Most Cancers

Aspirin has been studied as chemoprevention. The studies show mixed results but most have shown that aspirin does not prevent cancer. However, there is evidence that taking aspirin for long periods of time may prevent colorectal cancer in certain people. For more information, see Colorectal Cancer Prevention.

Results from a randomized trial suggest that taking aspirin may make cancer grow more quickly in the elderly, but longer follow up is needed to confirm these results.

Bleeding in the gastrointestinal tract or brain is a side effect of aspirin. Even though aspirin has not been shown to reduce the risk of most cancers, it has many uses, including helping to lower the chances of dying from heart disease. Before beginning long-term aspirin use, it is important to talk with your doctor about the related benefits and harms.

Vitamin and Dietary Supplements Have Not Been Shown to Prevent Cancer

An intervention is a treatment or action taken to prevent or treat disease, or improve health in other ways.

There is not enough proof that taking multivitamin and mineral supplements or single vitamins or minerals can prevent cancer. The following vitamins and mineral supplements have been studied, but have not been shown to lower the risk of cancer:

- Vitamin B6.
- Vitamin B12.
- Vitamin E.
- Vitamin C.
- Beta carotene.
- Folic acid.
- Selenium.
- Vitamin D.

The Selenium and Vitamin E Cancer Prevention Trial (SELECT) found that vitamin E taken alone increased the risk of prostate cancer. The risk continued even after the men stopped taking vitamin E. Taking selenium with vitamin E or taking selenium alone did not increase the risk of prostate cancer.

Vitamin D has also been studied to see if it has anticancer effects. Skin exposed to sunshine can make vitamin D. Vitamin D can also be consumed in the diet and in dietary supplements. Taking vitamin D in doses from 400–1100 IU/ day has not been shown to lower or increase the risk of cancer.

The VITamin D and OmegA-3 TriaL (VITAL) is under way to study whether taking vitamin D (2000 IU/ day) and omega-3 fatty acids from marine (oily fish) sources lowers the risk of cancer.

The Physicians' Health Study found that men who have had cancer in the past and take a multivitamin daily may have a slightly lower risk of having a second cancer.

See the following PDQ summaries for more information:

- Breast Cancer Prevention
- Colorectal Cancer Prevention
- Lung Cancer Prevention

- Prostate Cancer Prevention

New Ways to Prevent Cancer Are Being Studied in Clinical Trials

Information about clinical trials supported by NCI can be found on NCI's clinical trials search webpage. Clinical trials supported by other organizations can be found on the ClinicalTrials.gov website.

About This PDQ Summary

About PDQ

Physician Data Query (PDQ) is the National Cancer Institute's (NCI's) comprehensive cancer information database. The PDQ database contains summaries of the latest published information on cancer prevention, detection, genetics, treatment, supportive care, and complementary and alternative medicine. Most summaries come in two versions. The health professional versions have detailed information written in technical language. The patient versions are written in easy-to-understand, nontechnical language. Both versions have cancer information that is accurate and up to date and most versions are also available in Spanish.

PDQ is a service of the NCI. The NCI is part of the National Institutes of Health (NIH). NIH is the federal government's center of biomedical research. The PDQ summaries are based on an independent review of the medical literature. They are not policy statements of the NCI or the NIH.

Purpose of This Summary

This PDQ cancer information summary has current information about cancer prevention. It is meant to inform and help patients, families, and caregivers. It does not give formal guidelines or recommendations for making decisions about health care.

Reviewers and Updates

Editorial Boards write the PDQ cancer information summaries and keep them up to date. These Boards are made up of experts in cancer treatment and other specialties related to cancer. The summaries are reviewed regularly and changes are made when there is new information. The date on each summary ("Updated") is the date of the most recent change.

The information in this patient summary was taken from the health professional version, which is reviewed regularly and updated as needed, by the PDQ Screening and Prevention Editorial Board.

Clinical Trial Information

A clinical trial is a study to answer a scientific question, such as whether one treatment is better than another. Trials are based on past studies and what has been learned in the laboratory. Each trial answers certain scientific questions in order to find new and better ways to help cancer patients. During treatment clinical trials, information is collected about the effects of a new treatment and how well it works. If a clinical trial shows that a new treatment is better than one currently being used, the new treatment may become "standard." Patients may want to think about taking part in a clinical trial. Some clinical trials are open only to patients who have not started treatment.

Clinical trials can be found online at NCI's website. For more information, call the Cancer Information Service (CIS), NCI's contact center, at 1-800-4-CANCER (1-800-422-6237).

Permission to Use This Summary

PDQ is a registered trademark. The content of PDQ documents can be used freely as text. It cannot be identified as an NCI PDQ cancer information summary unless the whole summary is shown and it is updated regularly. However, a user would be allowed to write a sentence such as "NCI's PDQ cancer information summary about breast cancer prevention states the risks in the following way: [include excerpt from the summary]."

The best way to cite this PDQ summary is:

PDQ® Screening and Prevention Editorial Board. PDQ Cancer Prevention Overview. Bethesda, MD: National Cancer Institute. Updated

<MM/DD/YYYY>. Available at: https://www.cancer.gov/about-cancer/causes-prevention/patient-prevention-overview-pdq.Accessed <MM/DD/YYYY>. [PMID: 26389424].

Images in this summary are used with permission of the author(s), artist, and/or publisher for use in the PDQ summaries only. If you want to use an image from a PDQ summary and you are not using the whole summary, you must get permission from the owner. It cannot be given by the National Cancer Institute. Information about using the images in this summary, along with many other images related to cancer can be found in Visuals Online. Visuals Online is a collection of more than 3,000 scientific images.

Chapter 3

Diagnosis and Staging*

National Cancer Institute

Cancer can cause many different symptoms. Most often these symptoms are not caused by cancer, but by benign tumors or other problems. If you have symptoms that last for a couple of weeks, your doctor will do a physical exam and order tests or other procedures to find out what is causing your symptoms.

If you do find out you have cancer, your doctor will order another set of tests or procedures to figure out its stage. Stage refers to the extent of your cancer and is based on factors such as how large the tumor is and if it has spread. Once your doctor knows the stage of your cancer, he will be able to suggest treatment and discuss your prognosis with you. Understanding your cancer and knowing what to expect can help you and your loved ones feel more in control and cope with your diagnosis.

Symptoms of Cancer

Cancer can cause many symptoms, but these symptoms are most often caused by illness, injury, benign tumors, or other problems. If you have symptoms that do not get better after a few weeks, see your doctor so that problems can be diagnosed and treated as early as possible. Often, cancer does not cause pain, so do not wait to feel pain before seeing a doctor.

To learn more about symptoms for a specific cancer, see the list of PDQ® cancer treatment summaries for adult and childhood cancers. Each summary includes detailed information about symptoms caused by a specific cancer.

---

* This is an edited, reformatted and augmented version of National Cancer Institute Publication.

In: Understanding Cancer
Editor: Angela C. Ray
ISBN: 979-8-89530-769-4

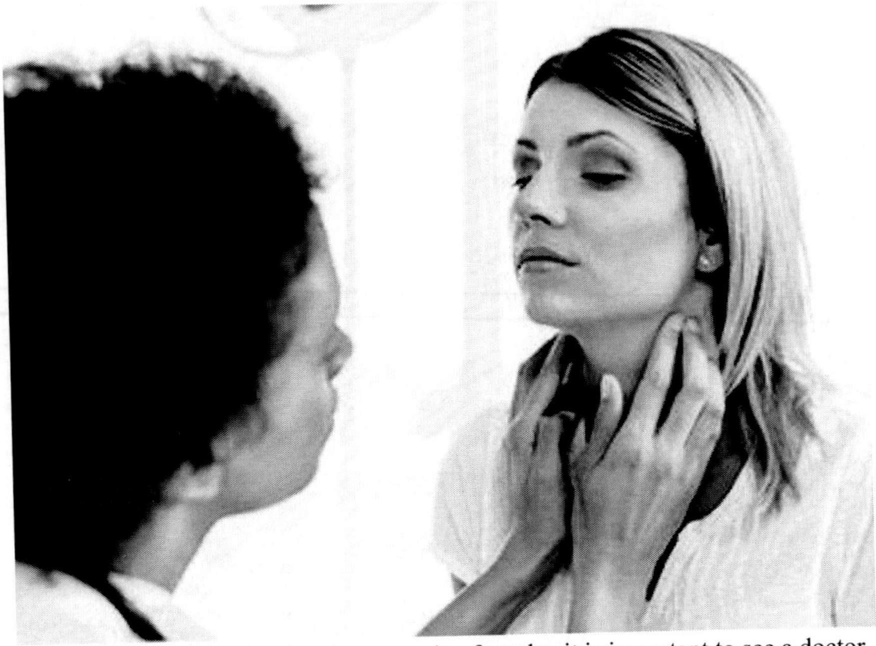

If you have symptoms that last for a couple of weeks, it is important to see a doctor. Credit: iStock.

Some of the symptoms that cancer may cause include:

Breast Changes

- Lump or firm feeling in your breast or under your arm
- Nipple changes or discharge
- Skin that is itchy, red, scaly, dimpled, or puckered

Bladder Changes

- Trouble urinating
- Pain when urinating
- Blood in the urine

Bleeding or Bruising, for No Known Reason

Bowel changes

- Blood in the stools
- Changes in bowel habits

Cough or Hoarseness That Does Not Go Away
Eating Problems

- Pain after eating (heartburn or indigestion that doesn't go away)
- Trouble swallowing
- Belly pain
- Nausea and vomiting
- Appetite changes

Fatigue That Is Severe and Lasts
Fever or Night Sweats for No Known Reason

Mouth changes

- A white or red patch on the tongue or in your mouth
- Bleeding, pain, or numbness in the lip or mouth

Neurological problems

- Headaches
- Seizures
- Vision changes
- Hearing changes
- Drooping of the face

Skin Changes

- A flesh-colored lump that bleeds or turns scaly

- A new mole or a change in an existing mole
- A sore that does not heal
- Jaundice (yellowing of the skin and whites of the eyes)

Swelling or Lumps Anywhere Such as in the Neck, Underarm, Stomach, and Groin
Weight Gain or Weight Loss for No Known Reason

How Cancer Is Diagnosed

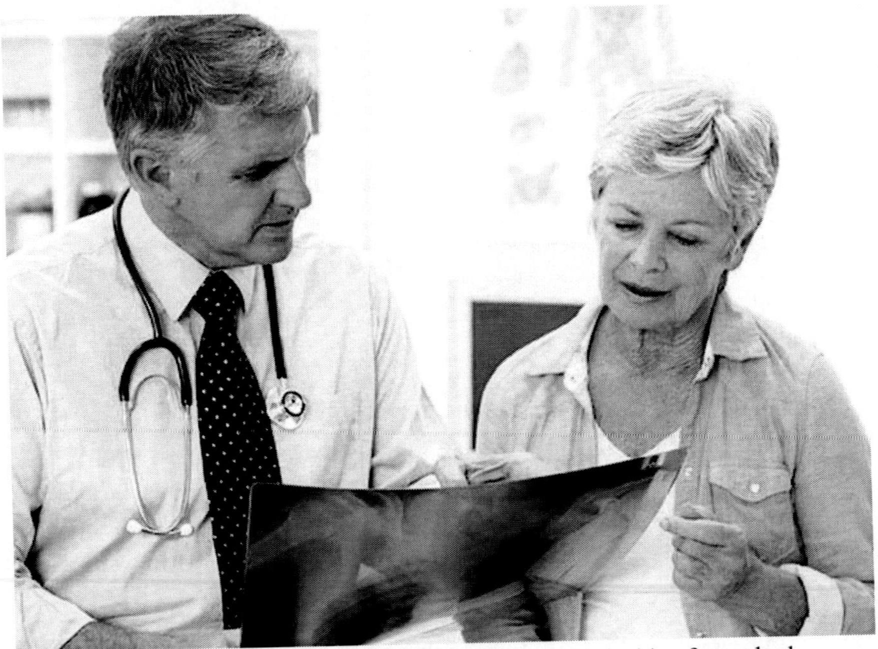

X-rays use low doses of radiation to create pictures of the inside of your body. Credit: iStock.

If you have a symptom or a screening test result that suggests cancer, your doctor will find out whether it is due to cancer or some other cause. There is no single test that can diagnose cancer. So your doctor may start by asking about your personal and family medical history and doing a physical exam. They may order lab tests, imaging tests (scans), or other tests or procedures.

You may also need a biopsy, which is often the only way to tell for sure if you have cancer.

This page covers tests that are often used to help diagnose cancer. Depending on your symptoms, you may have other tests, too. To learn more about how specific cancers are diagnosed, see the PDQ cancer treatment summaries for adult and childhood cancers. These summaries include detailed information about and pictures of diagnostic tests and procedures for each specific type of cancer.

Making Sense of Test Results

Results from lab tests, imaging, and biopsies are often posted in your patient portal before your doctor can discuss them with you. It is normal to feel anxious and want to know right away what the results are and what they mean. But your doctor is the best person to explain the results from all your tests and what they mean for you.

Lab Tests Used to Diagnose Cancer

High or low levels of certain substances in your body can be a sign of cancer. So lab tests of your blood, urine, and other body fluids that measure these substances can help doctors make a diagnosis. However, abnormal lab results are not a sure sign of cancer. Lab test results are used along with the results of other tests, such as biopsies and imaging, to help diagnose and learn more about a person's cancer.

It is important to keep in mind that lab results for healthy people can vary from person to person. Reasons for these differences include age, sex, race, medical history, and general health. In fact, your own results can vary from day to day. Because normal results can bounce around a bit, they are often reported in a range, with lower and upper limits. These ranges are based on test results from large numbers of people who have been tested in the past.

For many tests, it is possible to have normal results even if you have cancer. And it is possible to have test results outside the normal range even if you are healthy. These are some of the reasons why lab tests alone can't say for sure if you have cancer or any other disease.

Your doctor is the best person to explain your lab test results and what they mean for you.

Some common types of lab tests used to help diagnose cancer are listed below.

Blood Chemistry Test

What it does: A blood chemistry test measures the amounts of certain substances that are released into the blood by the organs and tissues of the body. These substances include metabolites, electrolytes, fats, sugars, and proteins, including enzymes.

What it tells us: Blood chemistry tests give important information about how well your kidneys, liver, and other organs are working. High or low levels of some substances in the blood can be a sign of disease or treatment side effects.

Complete Blood Count (CBC)

What it does: The CBC measures the number of red blood cells, white blood cells, and platelets in your blood. It also measures the amount of hemoglobin (the protein that carries oxygen) in your blood, the amount of your blood that is made up of red blood cells (hematocrit), the size of your red blood cells, and the amount of hemoglobin in your red blood cells.

How it is used: The CBC is often part of a routine health check-up. It can help diagnose some cancers, especially leukemias. It is also used to monitor your health during and after treatment.

Cytogenetic Analysis

What it does: Cytogenetic analysis looks for changes in chromosomes in samples of tissue, blood, bone marrow, or amniotic fluid. Chromosome changes may include broken, missing, rearranged, or extra chromosomes. Changes in certain chromosomes may be a sign of a genetic condition or some types of cancer.

How it is used: Cytogenetic analysis may be used to help diagnose cancer, plan treatment, or find out how well treatment is working.

Immunophenotyping

What it does: Immunophenotyping uses antibodies to identify cells based on the types of antigens or markers on the surface of the cells. It is most often done on blood or bone marrow samples. But it may also be done on other body fluids or tissue samples.

How it is used: Immunophenotyping helps diagnose, stage, and monitor blood cancers and other blood disorders, such as leukemias, lymphomas, myelodysplastic syndromes, and myeloproliferative disorders.

Liquid Biopsy

What it does: Liquid biopsy is a test done on a sample of blood to look for cancer cells or pieces of DNA from tumor cells that are sometimes released into the blood.

How it is used: A liquid biopsy may help find cancer at an early stage. It may also be used to help plan treatment or to find out how well treatment is working or if cancer has come back.

Sputum Cytology

What it does: Sputum cytology looks for abnormal cells in sputum, which is mucus and other matter brought up from the lungs by coughing.

How it is used: Sputum cytology can help diagnose lung cancer.

Tumor Marker Tests

What they do: Tests for tumor markers measure substances that are produced by cancer cells or other cells of the body in response to cancer. Most tumor markers are made by both normal cells and cancer cells. But they are produced at much higher levels by cancer cells.

How they are used: Tumor markers can be used to help diagnose cancer, decide on treatment, measure how well treatment worked, and watch for signs that the cancer has returned.

Learn more about tumor markers.

Urinalysis

What it does: Urinalysis describes the color of urine and measures its contents, such as sugar, protein, red blood cells, and white blood cells.

How it is used: Urinalysis can help diagnose kidney cancer, bladder cancer, and rarer urothelial cancers.

Urine Cytology

What it does: Urine cytology finds disease by looking for abnormal cells shed from the urinary tract into the urine.

How it is used: Urine cytology helps diagnose kidney cancer, bladder cancer, and rarer urothelial cancers. After cancer treatment, it is used to watch for signs that cancer has returned.

Imaging Tests Used in Cancer

Imaging tests create pictures of areas inside your body that help the doctor see whether a tumor is present. These pictures can be made in several ways.

CT scan

A CT scan uses an x-ray machine linked to a computer to take a series of pictures of your organs from different angles. These pictures are used to create detailed 3-D images of the inside of your body.

Sometimes, you may receive a dye or other contrast material before you have the scan. You might swallow the dye, or it may be given by a needle into a vein. Contrast material helps make the pictures easier to read by highlighting certain areas in the body.

During the CT scan, you will lie still on a table that slides into a donut-shaped scanner. The CT machine moves around you, taking pictures.

Learn more about CT scans and how they are used to diagnose cancer.

MRI

An *MRI* uses a powerful magnet and radio waves to take pictures of your body in slices. These slices are combined to create detailed images of the inside of your body, which can show places where there may be tumors.

When you have an MRI, you lie still on a table that is pushed into a long chamber that surrounds part or all of your body. The MRI machine makes loud thumping noises and rhythmic beats.

Sometimes, you might have a special dye injected into your vein before or during your MRI exam. This dye, called a contrast agent, can make tumors show up brighter in the pictures.

Nuclear Scan

A nuclear scan uses radioactive material to take pictures of the inside of the body. This type of scan may also be called a radionuclide scan.

Before this scan, you receive an injection of a small amount of radioactive material, which is sometimes called a tracer. It flows through your bloodstream and collects in certain bones or organs.

During the scan, you lie still on a table while a machine called a scanner detects and measures the radioactivity in your body, creating pictures of bones or organs on a computer screen or on film.

After the scan, the radioactive material in your body will lose its radioactivity over time. It may also leave your body through your urine or stool.

Bone Scan

Bone scans are a type of nuclear scan that check for abnormal areas or damage in the bones. They may be used to diagnose bone cancer or find out whether cancer has spread to the bones from elsewhere in the body (called metastatic bone tumors).

Before this test, a very small amount of radioactive material is injected into your vein. As it travels through the blood, the material collects in abnormal areas in the bone. Areas where the material collects show up on pictures taken by a special scanner. These areas are called "hot spots."

PET Scan

A PET scan is a type of nuclear scan that makes detailed 3-D pictures of areas inside your body where glucose is taken up. Because cancer cells often take up more glucose than healthy cells, the pictures can be used to find cancer in the body.

Before the scan, you receive an injection of a tracer called radioactive glucose. During the scan, you will lie still on a table that moves back and forth through a scanner.

Ultrasound

An ultrasound exam uses high-energy sound waves that people cannot hear. The sound waves echo off tissues inside your body. A computer uses these echoes to create pictures of areas inside your body. This picture is called a sonogram.

During an ultrasound exam, you will lie on a table while a technologist slowly moves a device called a transducer, which makes the high-energy sound waves, on the skin over the part of the body that is being examined. The transducer is covered with a warm gel that helps it glide over the skin.

X-rays

X-rays use low doses of radiation to create pictures inside your body. An x-ray technologist will put you in position and direct the x-ray beam to the correct part of your body. While the images are taken, you will need to stay very still and may need to hold your breath for a second or two.

Biopsy

In most cases, doctors need to do a biopsy to be certain that you have cancer. A biopsy is a procedure in which the doctor removes a sample of abnormal tissue. A pathologist looks at the tissue under a microscope and runs other tests on the cells in the sample. The pathologist describes the findings in a pathology report, which contains details about your diagnosis. The information in your pathology reports can also help show what treatment options might work for you.

Learn more about pathology reports and the type of information they contain.

The biopsy sample may be obtained in several ways.

With a needle: The doctor uses a needle to withdraw tissue or fluid. This method is used for bone marrow aspirations, spinal taps, and some breast, prostate, and liver biopsies.

With endoscopy: The doctor inserts a thin, lighted tube called an endoscope into a natural body opening, such as the mouth or anus. The doctor can remove some or all of the abnormal tissue through the endoscope.

Examples of endoscopy exams include:

- Colonoscopy, which is an exam of the colon and rectum. In this type of exam, an endoscope goes through the anus.
- Bronchoscopy, which is an exam of the trachea, bronchi, and lungs. In this type of exam, an endoscope goes through the mouth or nose and down the throat.

With surgery: A surgeon removes an area of abnormal cells during an operation. Surgery may be excisional or incisional.

In an excisional biopsy, the surgeon removes the entire area of abnormal cells. Often some of the normal tissue around these cells is also removed.

In an incisional biopsy, the surgeon removes just part of the abnormal area.

Some biopsies may require a sedative or anesthesia.

Sedatives are medicine that helps you relax and stay very still or sleep during a biopsy.

Anesthesia keeps you from feeling pain. It refers to drugs or other substances that cause you to lose feeling or awareness. There are three types of anesthesia.

- *local anesthesia*, which causes loss of feeling in one small area of the body
- *regional anesthesia*, which causes loss of feeling in a part of the body, such as an arm or leg
- *general anesthesia,* which causes loss of feeling and a complete loss of awareness that seems like a very deep sleep

What Happens If Tests Show You Have Cancer

If the biopsy and other tests show that you have cancer, you may have more tests to help your doctor plan treatment. For instance, your doctor may do other tests to figure out if the cancer has spread and how far. This information is important for knowing the stage of your cancer. For some cancers, other pathology studies are done to find out the grade of the tumor. Or tumor markers are studied to find out the risk group that you fall into. This information is important for deciding on the best treatment. Your tumor may also be tested further for other tumor markers or biomarkers.

To learn more about the diagnosis, staging, and treatment for your type of cancer, see the PDQ cancer treatment summaries for adult and childhood cancers.

Tumor Grade

Tumor grade describes how normal or abnormal cancer cells look under a microscope. The more normal the cells look, the less aggressive the cancer and the more slowly it grows and spreads. On the other hand, the more abnormal the cells look, the more aggressive the cancer and the faster it is likely to grow and spread.

Tumor grade is not the same thing as cancer stage. Stage refers to how large a cancer tumor is and how far the cancer has spread. See Cancer Staging to learn more.

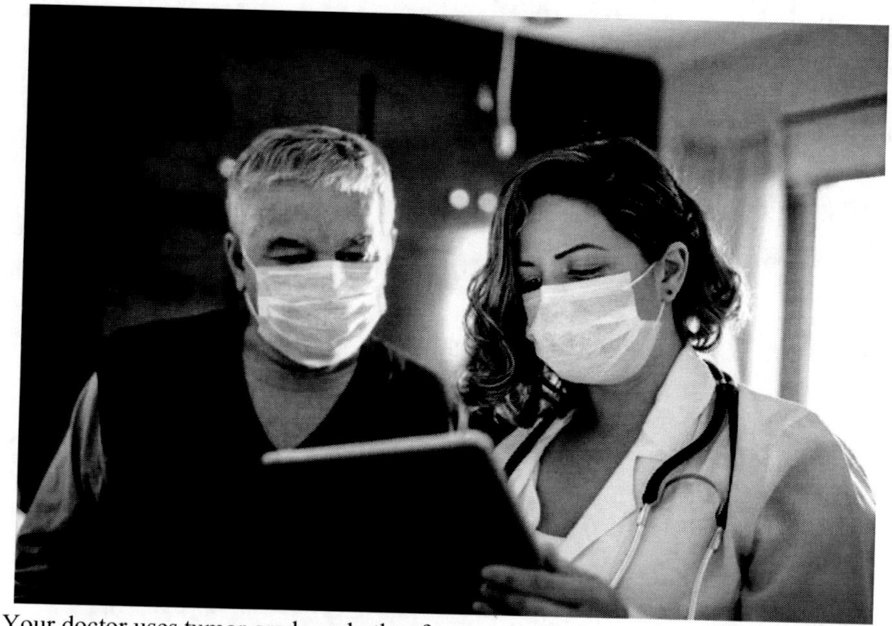

Your doctor uses tumor grade and other factors about your cancer to form a treatment plan and in some cases, to estimate your prognosis.
Credit: iStock.

How Tumor Grade Is Determined

In most cases, doctors need to study a sample of tissue from the tumor to decide if it is cancer and, if it is, its grade. They obtain this tissue by doing a biopsy, a procedure in which they remove all or part of the tumor. A specialist called a pathologist determines the grade of your tumor by studying samples from the biopsy under a microscope. The pathologist describes the findings in a pathology report, which also contains other details about your diagnosis.

Cells that look more normal might be called well-differentiated in the pathology report. And cells that look less normal might be called poorly differentiated or undifferentiated. Based on these and other features of how cells look under the microscope, the pathologist will assign a number to describe the grade.

Different factors are used to decide the grade of different cancers. To learn about the factors that go into deciding the grade of your cancer, find your type of cancer in the PDQ® cancer treatment summaries for adult and childhood cancers.

How Tumor Grade Is Described

Systems for describing tumor grade can differ depending on the type of cancer. But most tumors are graded as X, 1, 2, 3, or 4.

- Grade X: Grade cannot be assessed (undetermined grade)
- Grade 1: Well differentiated (low grade)
- Grade 2: Moderately differentiated (intermediate grade)
- Grade 3: Poorly differentiated (high grade)
- Grade 4: Undifferentiated (high grade)

In grade 1 tumors, the cells look close to normal. The higher the number, the more abnormal the cells look. Grade 4 tumors look most abnormal.

To learn more about the system that describes tumor grade for your cancer, see the PDQ® cancer treatment summaries for adult and childhood cancers.

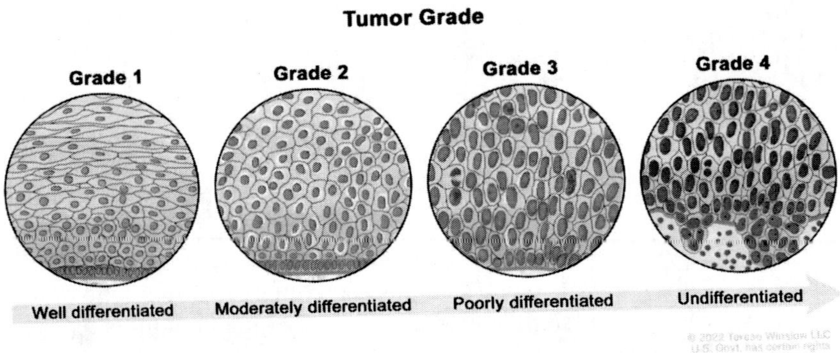

Tumor grade describes how normal or abnormal cancer cells look under a microscope. The higher the grade, the more abnormal the cells look and the faster it is likely to grow and spread.
Credit: © Terese Winslow.

How Tumor Grade Affects Your Treatment Options

Your doctor uses tumor grade and other factors about your cancer to form a treatment plan and in some cases, to estimate your prognosis. Prognosis is an estimate of how the disease will likely go for you. Other factors that go into deciding on a treatment plan include cancer stage, genetic features of the tumor, your age, and your general health. Since a high-grade cancer may grow and spread more quickly, it may require more aggressive treatment right away.

To learn about treatment for your cancer, see the PDQ® cancer treatment summaries for adult and childhood cancers for your type of cancer.

Tumor Markers

What Are Tumor Markers?

A tumor marker is anything present in or produced by cancer cells or other cells of the body in response to cancer or certain benign (noncancerous) conditions that provides information about a cancer, such as how aggressive it is, what kind of treatment it may respond to, or whether it is responding to treatment.

Tumor markers have traditionally been proteins or other substances that are made at higher amounts by cancer cells than normal cells. These can be found in the blood, urine, stool, tumors, or other tissues or bodily fluids of some patients with cancer.

Increasingly, however, genomic markers (such as tumor gene mutations, patterns of tumor gene expression, and nongenetic changes in tumor DNA) are being used as tumor markers. These markers are found both in tumors themselves and in tumor fragments shed into bodily fluids.

Many different tumor markers have been characterized and are in clinical use. Some are associated with only one type of cancer, whereas others are associated with multiple cancer types.

How Are Tumor Markers Used in Cancer Care?

Tumor markers can provide a wide variety of information that is important for cancer care, such as

- Helping to diagnose cancer. However, having an elevated level of a tumor marker does not mean that someone has cancer. Noncancerous conditions can sometimes cause an increase in the level of a tumor marker. In addition, not everyone with a particular type of cancer will have a higher level of a tumor marker associated with that cancer. Therefore, measurements of tumor markers are usually combined with the results of other tests, such as biopsies or imaging, to diagnose cancer.

- The type of cancer
- The stage of the cancer
- An estimate of prognosis
- What treatment may be effective. Tumor markers that indicate whether someone is a candidate for a particular targeted therapy are sometimes referred to as biomarkers for cancer treatment. Biomarkers are generally measured in samples of tumor tissue. However, tumors can shed cells or bits of biological material into blood, and these can be measured by tests called liquid biopsies.
- How well the treatment is working. Periodic (or "serial") measurements of a marker made while someone is undergoing treatment can indicate whether the tumor is responding to treatment.
- Whether cancer has returned. Measuring tumor markers periodically after treatment has ended may be used to check for recurrence.

What Tumor Marker Tests Are Currently Being Used, and for Which Cancer Types?

A number of tumor marker tests are currently being used for a wide range of cancer types. See the list of tumor marker tests in common use for more information.

Many tumor marker tests are carried out by commercial and academic laboratories. Sometimes cancer centers use a tumor marker test developed within a single clinical laboratory (also known as a lab-developed test or LDT) to meet a specific medical need. All tumor markers, including those tested by LDTs, are tested in laboratories that meet standards set by the Clinical Laboratory Improvement Amendments program.

Can Tumor Markers Be Used to Detect Cancer in People Who Don't Have Symptoms?

Because tumors produce markers that can be measured in blood and other body fluids, researchers have hoped that they might also be useful in screening people for cancer—that is, detecting cancer at an early stage before it causes symptoms.

However, studies to see whether circulating tumor markers can be used to screen for cancer have generally found that these markers do not work well for screening. They often don't identify everyone with the disease (they are not sensitive enough). Or they may indicate the possible presence of cancer in people who don't actually have cancer (they are not specific enough).

Researchers are now testing whether multi-cancer detection tests (MCDs), which analyze multiple biomarkers in the blood of people without symptoms, can identify early cancers.

Most MCDs examine DNA that tumor cells release into blood. They may also analyze other biological molecules in blood, such as proteins. Tests that look at tumor markers in blood and other body fluids are sometimes called liquid biopsy tests.

Although many MCD tests are in development and several are already being marketed, much remains to be learned about how best to use these tests and their harms and benefits. A critical question is whether treating the cancers identified by MCD tests would reduce deaths from these cancers. NCI will be launching a clinical trial to better understand the implications of using MCD tests to screen for cancer.

What Research Is Under Way to Develop Additional Tumor Markers?

NCI's Early Detection Research Network (EDRN), a collaborative consortium of academic and private-sector investigators, has focused on the systematic discovery, development, and validation of biomarkers and imaging methods to detect early-stage cancers and to assess risk for developing cancer. One goal of EDRN is to develop biomarkers that can distinguish aggressive early-stage cancers from slow-growing cancers that would never cause symptoms to reduce overtreatment.

Cancer researchers are turning to proteomics (the study of protein structure, function, and patterns of expression) and proteogenomics (the integration of proteomics with genomics and gene expression analysis, or transcriptomics) with the hope of developing novel biomarkers that can be used to identify cancer in its early stages, to predict the effectiveness of treatment, and to predict the chance of cancer recurrence.

Artificial intelligence and machine learning are increasingly being investigated, including by EDRN, as tools to analyze and interpret patterns in genomic and proteomic markers that help predict cancer risk and diagnose specific cancer types.

NCI's Clinical Proteomic Tumor Analysis Consortium (CPTAC) is using a proteogenomic approach for tumor marker discovery for a growing number of cancers, including colorectal, breast, and ovarian cancers. By systematically identifying proteins (and associated biological processes) that originate from alterations in cancer genomes, CPTAC researchers have discovered new tumor subtypes, tumor microenvironment variations, and new potential proteins for targeted drug therapy. Recent innovations have suggested that these analyses could be done on a microscale using very small amounts of tumor tissue obtain from a biopsy.

The NCI Cancer Moonshot^{SM} Biobank is working with patient participants at community hospitals around the country to encourage them to donate tissue and blood samples over the course of their cancer treatment. The samples are sent to researchers who use them to better understand cancer and potentially identify tumor markers.

More information on NCI's role in supporting research on novel tools and methods for diagnosing cancer is available on the Cancer Diagnosis Research page.

Selected References

1) Bettegowda C, Sausen M, Leary RJ, et al. Detection of circulating tumor DNA in early- and late-stage human malignancies. *Science Translational Medicine* 2014; 6(224):224ra24.
[PubMed Abstract]

2) Duffy MJ. Clinical uses of tumor markers: a critical review. *Critical Reviews in Clinical Laboratory Sciences* 2001; 38(3):225–262.
[PubMed Abstract]

3) Duffy MJ. Tumor markers in clinical practice: A review focusing on common solid cancers. *Medical Principles and Practice* 2013; 22(1):4–11.
[PubMed Abstract]
4) Lennon AM, Buchanan AH, Kinde I, et al. Feasibility of blood testing combined with PET-CT to screen for cancer and guide intervention. *Science* 2020; 369(6499):eabb9601.
[PubMed Abstract]
5) Springer SU, Chen CH, Rodriguez Pena MDC, et al. Non-invasive detection of urothelial cancer through the analysis of driver gene mutations and aneuploidy. *Elife* 2018; 7:e32143.
[PubMed Abstract]
6) Wang Y, Li L, Douville C, et al. Evaluation of liquid from the Papanicolaou test and other liquid biopsies for the detection of endometrial and ovarian cancers. *Science Translational Medicine* 2018; 10(433):eaap8793.
[PubMed Abstract]

Pathology Reports

What is a pathology report?

A pathology report (sometimes called a surgical pathology report) is a medical report that describes the characteristics of a tissue specimen that is taken from a patient. The pathology report is written by a pathologist, a doctor who has special training in identifying diseases by studying cells and tissues under a microscope.

A pathology report includes identifying information (such as the patient's name, birthdate, and biopsy date) and details about where in the body the specimen is from and how it was obtained. It typically includes a gross description (a visual description of the specimen as seen by the naked eye), a microscopic description, and a final diagnosis. It may also include a section for comments by the pathologist.

The pathology report provides the definitive cancer diagnosis. It is also used for staging (describing the extent of cancer within the body, especially whether it has spread) and to help plan treatment.

Common terms that may appear on a cancer pathology report include:

- invasive
- noninvasive
- in situ
- carcinoma
- benign
- neoplasm
- malignant
- adenocarcinoma
- margin
- infiltrating
- ductal
- undifferentiated
- well-differentiated

How Is Tissue Obtained for Examination by a Pathologist?

The pathologist examines cells or tissues obtained during a biopsy (which is a procedure to remove a cell or tissue specimen for examination by a pathologist) or surgery or from bodily fluids.

A biopsy specimen can be obtained in several ways, such as by

- taking a tissue sample from the surface of the skin
- using a needle inserted through the skin to withdraw tissue or fluid
- inserting a thin, lighted tube called an endoscope through the mouth, anus, urethra, or a small incision in the skin to look at areas inside the body and remove a sample using special tools that pass through the tube

If surgery is used to remove part or all of a tumor, some or all of the removed tumor specimen will be examined by the pathologist. If the entire tumor is removed, typically the surgeon will attempt to remove some normal tissue around the tumor (known as the margin) for examination by the pathologist to make sure that it doesn't contain tumor cells.

For some cancer types, especially breast cancer and melanoma, the surgeon may also remove nearby lymph nodes, called the sentinel lymph nodes, so the pathologist can see if these contain cancer cells. The Sentinel

Lymph Node Biopsy fact sheet describes this procedure and its use in determining the extent, or stage, of cancer in the body.

A pathologist may also examine cells that are present in bodily fluids, such as urine, cerebrospinal fluid (the fluid around the brain and spinal cord), sputum (mucus from the lungs), peritoneal (abdominal cavity) fluid, pleural (chest cavity) fluid, cervical/vaginal smears, and bone marrow.

How Does a Pathologist Examine Tissue?

Tissue or cell specimens must be cut into very thin slices, called sections, so the pathologist can look at them under a microscope. The specimen must be processed to make it solid before it can be cut into sections.

The most common approach used for tissue examination involves chemically "fixing" the specimen, usually with a chemical called formalin. This stabilizes the cells for further processing in an automated machine that submerges the tissue in substances that remove water and replace it with molten paraffin wax.

Once processed, the tissue is embedded into a permanent paraffin wax block to be cut. The paraffin-embedded tissue is then sliced into very thin sections that are placed onto microscopic slides. The slides are stained with dyes to help visualize parts of the cell and structures in the tissue. This is known as histologic (tissue) examination.

Fixed sections provide the maximum detail of the structures in a tissue sample, and they can be saved and analyzed in the future if needed. Preparing fixed sections normally takes several days. The pathologist typically sends a pathology report to the doctor within 10 days after the biopsy or surgery is performed.

Frozen sectioning is another approach used by a pathologist for tissue examination. Frozen sections are prepared when an immediate answer about a tissue sample is needed. For example, this type of examination would be used during surgery to provide the surgeon with a rapid diagnosis for an area of abnormal tissue and the extent of the abnormal area while the patient is in the operating room. To make frozen sections, the tissue sample is rapidly frozen, cut into sections using an instrument called a cryostat, stained, and examined by a pathologist. This can be done in about 15 to 20 minutes.

Frozen sections are suitable for preparing tissue for some tests, such as immunofluorescence and *immunohistochemistry*. However, the fixed (permanent) section preserves more detail and is more commonly used to make a diagnosis than frozen sections.

What Is the Gross Description on a Surgical Pathology Report?

The gross description includes the color, weight, and size of a tissue sample as seen by the naked eye. It may also include the shape of the tissue sample and any visible abnormalities. And it will indicate the body site from where the tissue was taken from, how many samples were taken, and whether and how many lymph nodes were removed.

What Is the Microscopic Description on a Surgical Pathology Report?

The microscopic description in a pathology report includes information about the appearance of the cells after they have been stained with routine stains such as hematoxylin and eosin (also known as H&E) and viewed under the microscope. H&E staining helps identify different types of cells and tissues and provides important information about the pattern and shape of cells and the structure of the tissue. With H&E staining, hematoxylin shows the ribosomes, chromatin (genetic material) within the nucleus, and some other structures in the nucleus as a deep blue-purple color. Eosin shows the cytoplasm, collagen, connective tissue, and other structures that surround and support the cell as an orange-pink-red color.

This description may also include the type and number of cells seen in the tissue sample, how abnormal the cells look (also called the tumor grade), and whether there are notable cell features (such as their arrangement and behavior).

The microscopic description section will also indicate whether abnormal cells are found in the margins (the edges of the tissue that has been removed by surgery) or in lymph nodes. Margins are described as negative (or "clean") when the pathologist finds no cancer cells at the edge of the tissue, suggesting that all of the cancer has been removed. A margin is described as positive (or "involved") when the pathologist finds cancer cells at the edge of the tissue, suggesting that some of the cancer has not been removed. Lymph nodes are called positive if they have cancer cells and negative if they do not.

This description may also include the results of additional tests that were performed on the tissue. Depending on the cancer type, these may include tests that

- measure the properties of cells in a sample, including the number of cells, percentage of live cells, cell size and shape, and the proportion of cells that have a tumor marker on their cell surface. See NCI's Tumor Markers fact sheet for more information about tumor markers and how they are used in cancer diagnosis and treatment.
- investigate genetic or molecular abnormalities in specimens with the use of specific techniques. These include karyotyping, to detect aneuploidy (abnormal numbers of chromosomes) and large translocations (in which long pieces of chromosomes have broken off and moved to other chromosomes), as well as fluorescence in situ hybridization, to detect specific chromosomal deletions or translocations.

What Is the Diagnosis on a Surgical Pathology Report?

The diagnosis section of a pathology report is the pathologist's summary of all the findings of their visual and microscopic examination of the tissue specimen, in combination with relevant clinical information. It is in this section that the cancer type will be identified, including the tumor grade, lymph node status, margin status, and stage.

Are Molecular Characteristics of a Tumor Included on a Surgical Pathology Report?

Certain molecular tests, sometimes called biomarker tests, are done as part of the initial pathology analysis for all cases of a given cancer type. For example, a pathology report for a patient with suspected breast cancer will include the results of testing for estrogen and progesterone receptors and the protein HER2/neu. The results of these tests can help identify what treatments are best for an individual patient.

A liquid biopsy—in which a sample of blood or other body fluid is tested to look for pieces of DNA that have been released from tumor cells—is another way that the molecular characteristics of a tumor may be analyzed. The findings of these additional tests may be provided in separate reports that are linked to the pathology report.

Pathology examination is increasingly incorporating analyses of the structure and sequence of DNA extracted from fresh and fixed tissue samples to refine the cancer diagnosis through improved subtyping and stratification of tumor types and to better inform treatment.

What Other Information Might Be Included on a Surgical Pathology Report?

In the comments section of the pathology report, the pathologist may note unusual features of the sample, such as information about the cytogenetic and/or molecular characteristics of a tumor, or provide additional information. The comments section is often used by the pathologist to provide more details about the disease and its diagnosis and to recommend additional tests that might be needed. It may include relevant clinical history or test results, abnormal findings that could change a typical diagnosis, previous samples or diagnoses for the patient, and other possible diagnoses. It will also mention tests that are still in process (i.e., pending).

How Will I Find Out What's in My Surgical Pathology Report?

The doctor in charge of a patient's treatment will tell the patient about the findings in the pathology report and can help the patient understand the report and what it means for their situation. A patient can also ask to discuss their report with the pathologist.

Patients should be aware that pathology report results will often appear in the patient portal at the same time the doctor receives them. This means that patients may see their report before their doctor has had a chance to review it and discuss it with them.

Can Individuals Get a Second Opinion on Their Surgical Pathology Results?

Although the diagnosis of most cancers is straightforward, patients or their doctors may want to get a second opinion from another pathologist. Patients interested in getting a second opinion should talk with their doctor. They will need to obtain the slides and/or paraffin block from the pathologist who examined the sample or from the hospital where the biopsy or surgery was done.

Many institutions provide second opinions on pathology specimens. NCI-designated cancer centers or academic institutions sometimes provide second opinions. Patients should contact the facility in advance to determine if this service is available, the cost, and shipping instructions.

For each patient, the results of all pathology examinations and any other tests ordered by the pathologists are reviewed together by the tumor review board, a group of doctors who are experts in different specialties who plan the treatment approach for a patient.

Cancer Staging

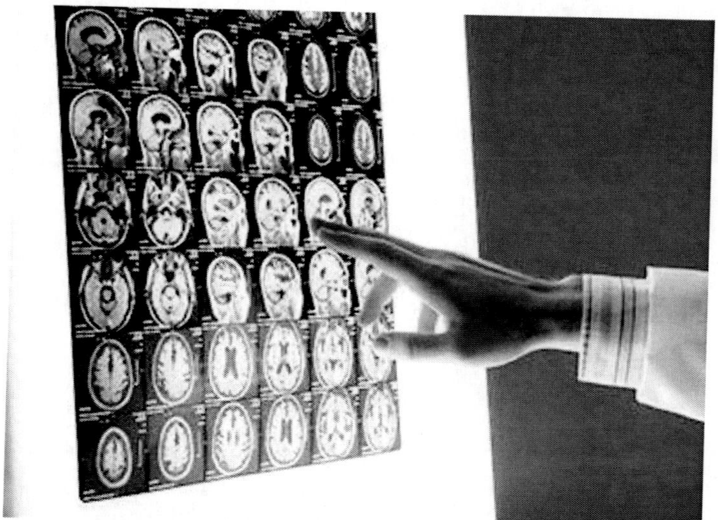

To learn the stage of your disease, your doctor may order x-rays, lab tests, and other tests or procedures.
Credit: Veer.

Stage refers to the extent of your cancer, such as how large the tumor is and if it has spread. Knowing the stage of your cancer helps your doctor

- understand how serious your cancer is and your chances of survival
- plan the best treatment for you
- identify clinical trials that may be treatment options for you

A cancer is always referred to by the stage it was given at diagnosis, even if it gets worse or spreads. New information about how a cancer has changed over time is added to the original stage. So the stage doesn't change, even though the cancer might.

How Stage Is Determined

To learn the stage of your disease, your doctor may order x-rays, lab tests, and other tests or procedures. See the section on How Cancer Is Diagnosed to learn more about these tests.

Systems That Describe Stage

There are many staging systems. Some, such as the TNM staging system, are used for many types of cancer. Others are specific to a particular type of cancer. Most staging systems include information about

- where the tumor is located in the body
- the size of the tumor
- whether the cancer has spread to nearby lymph nodes
- whether the cancer has spread to a different part of the body

The TNM Staging System

The TNM system is the most widely used cancer staging system. Most hospitals and medical centers use the TNM system as their main method for cancer reporting. You are likely to see your cancer described by this staging system in your pathology report unless there is a different staging system for your type of cancer. Examples of cancers with different staging systems include brain and spinal cord tumors and blood cancers.

In the TNM system

- The T refers to the size and extent of the main tumor. The main tumor is usually called the primary tumor.
- The N refers to the number of nearby lymph nodes that have cancer.
- The M refers to whether the cancer has metastasized. This means that the cancer has spread from the primary tumor to other parts of the body.

When your cancer is described by the TNM system, there will be numbers after each letter that give more details about the cancer—for example, T1N0MX or T3N1M0. The following explains what the letters and numbers mean.

Primary tumor (T)

- TX: Main tumor cannot be measured.
- T0: Main tumor cannot be found.
- T1, T2, T3, T4: Refers to the size and/or extent of the main tumor. The higher the number after the T, the larger the tumor or the more it has grown into nearby tissues. T's may be further divided to provide more detail, such as T3a and T3b.

Regional lymph nodes (N)

- NX: Cancer in nearby lymph nodes cannot be measured.
- N0: There is no cancer in nearby lymph nodes.
- N1, N2, N3: Refers to the number and location of lymph nodes that contain cancer. The higher the number after the N, the more lymph nodes that contain cancer.

Distant metastasis (M)

- MX: Metastasis cannot be measured.
- M0: Cancer has not spread to other parts of the body.
- M1: Cancer has spread to other parts of the body

Other Ways to Describe Stage

The TNM system helps describe cancer in great detail. But for many cancers, the TNM combinations are grouped into five less-detailed stages. The following chart shows how your doctor or nurse may describe your cancer.

Stage	What it means
Stage 0	Abnormal cells are present but have not spread to nearby tissue. Also called carcinoma in situ, or CIS. CIS is not cancer, but it may become cancer.
Stage I, Stage II, and Stage III (may also be written as Stage 1, Stage 2, and Stage 3)	Cancer is present. The higher the number, the larger the cancer tumor and the more it has spread into nearby tissues.
Stage IV (may also be written as Stage 4)	The cancer has spread to distant parts of the body.

The higher the number, the more advanced the cancer is. Letters and numbers are often used after the first number to describe the cancer in more detail. For instance, Stage 2 prostate cancer may be further divided into 2A, 2B, or 2C.

Another staging system that is used for all types of cancer groups cancer into one of five main categories. This staging system is more often used by cancer registries than by doctors. But you may still hear your doctor or nurse describe your cancer in one of the following ways.

- *In situ*—Abnormal cells are present but have not spread to nearby tissue.
- *Localized*—Cancer is limited to the place where it started, with no sign that it has spread.
- *Regional*—Cancer has spread to nearby lymph nodes, tissues, or organs.
- *Distant*—Cancer has spread to distant parts of the body.
- *Unknown*—There is not enough information to figure out the stage.

To learn more about staging for your type of cancer, see the PDQ® cancer treatment summaries for adult and childhood cancers.

Understanding Cancer Prognosis

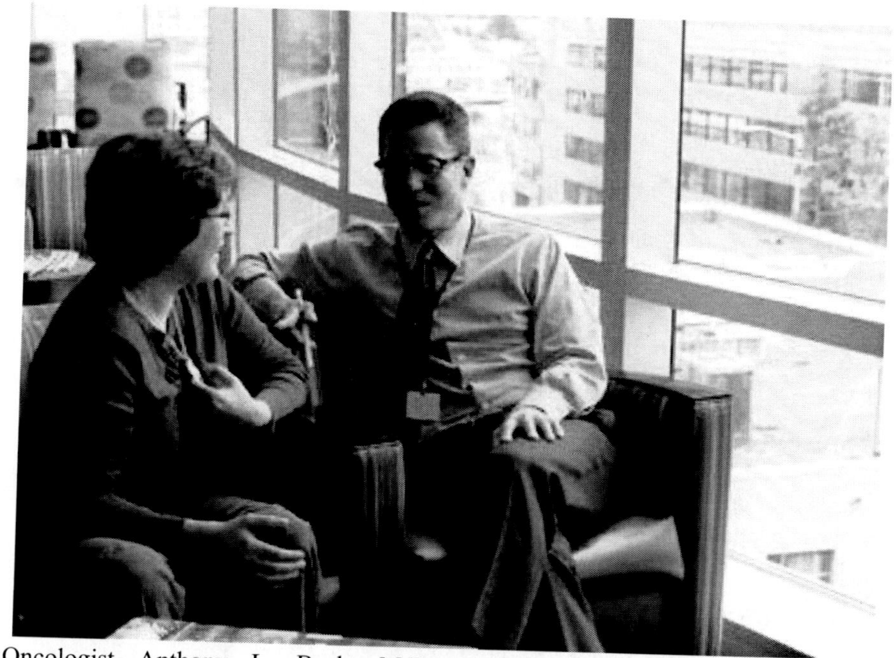

Oncologist Anthony L. Back, M.D., a national expert on doctor-patient communications, talks with one of his patients about what she'd like to know of her prognosis.
Credit: National Cancer Institute.

If you have cancer, you may have questions about how serious your cancer is and your chances of survival. The estimate of how the disease will go for you is called prognosis. It can be hard to understand what prognosis means and also hard to talk about, even for

Factors That Can Affect Your Prognosis

Some of the factors that affect prognosis include:

- the type of cancer and where it is in your body
- the stage of the cancer, which refers to the size of the cancer and if it has spread to other parts of your body

- the cancer's grade, which refers to how abnormal the cancer cells look under a microscope and provides clues about how quickly the cancer is likely to grow and spread
- certain traits of the cancer cells, such as certain genetic changes or hormone receptor status
- your age and how healthy you were before cancer
- how you respond to treatment

Learn more about Cancer Staging and Tumor Grade.

Seeking Information About Your Prognosis Is a Personal Decision

When you have cancer, you and your loved ones face many unknowns. Understanding your cancer and knowing what to expect can help you and your loved ones make decisions. Some of the decisions you may face include:

- Which treatment is best for you?
- If you want treatment?
- How to best take care of yourself and manage treatment side effects?
- How to deal with financial and legal matters?

Many people want to know their prognosis. They find it easier to cope when they know more about their cancer. You may ask your doctor about survival statistics or search for this information on your own. Or you may find statistics confusing and frightening, and think they are too impersonal to be of value to you. It is up to you to decide how much information you want.

If you do decide you want to know more, the doctor who knows the most about your situation is in the best position to discuss your prognosis and explain what the statistics may mean.

If you need help coping with your prognosis, you may find our information on Coping with Cancer helpful.

Understanding Statistics About Survival

Doctors estimate prognosis by using statistics that researchers have collected over many years about people with the same type of cancer. Several types of statistics may be used to estimate prognosis. The most commonly used statistics include:

- *Cancer-specific survival*
  This is the percentage of people with a specific type and stage of cancer who have not died from their cancer during a certain period of time after diagnosis. The period of time may be 1 year, 2 years, 5 years, etc., with 5 years being the time period most often used. Cancer-specific survival is also called disease-specific survival. In most cases, cancer-specific survival is based on causes of death listed in medical records.
- *Relative survival*
  This statistic is another method used to estimate cancer-specific survival that does not use information about the cause of death. It is the percentage of people with cancer who have survived for a certain period of time after diagnosis compared to people who do not have cancer.
- *Overall survival*
  This is the percentage of people with a specific type and stage of cancer who have not died from any cause during a certain period of time after diagnosis.
- *Disease-free survival*
  This statistic is the percentage of patients who have no signs of cancer during a certain period of time after treatment. Other names for this statistic are recurrence-free or progression-free survival.

Because statistics are based on large groups of people, they cannot be used to predict exactly what will happen to you. Everyone is different. Treatments and how people respond to treatment can differ greatly. Also, it takes years to see the benefit of new treatments and ways of finding cancer. So, the statistics your doctor uses to make a prognosis may not be based on treatments being used today.

Still, your doctor may tell you that you have a good prognosis if statistics suggest that your cancer is likely to respond well to treatment. Or they may tell you that you have a poor prognosis if the cancer is harder to control. Whatever your doctor tells you, keep in mind that a prognosis is an educated guess. Your doctor cannot be certain how it will go for you.

Where to Find Cancer Statistics

NCI collects and reports on cancer statistics through its SEER Program, which stands for Surveillance, Epidemiology, and End Results. From the Cancer Stat Facts page on the SEER web site, you can find answers to the most commonly asked questions about cancer statistics for many cancer types. You can also browse the latest SEER Cancer Statistics Review.

If You Decide Not to Have Treatment

If you decide not to have treatment, the doctor who knows your situation best is in the best position to discuss your prognosis.

Survival statistics most often come from studies that compare treatments with each other, rather than treatment with no treatment. So, it may not be easy for your doctor to give you an accurate prognosis.

Understanding the Difference Between Cure and Remission

Cure means that there are no traces of your cancer after treatment and the cancer will never come back.

Remission means that the signs and symptoms of your cancer are reduced. Remission can be partial or complete. In a complete remission, all signs and symptoms of cancer have disappeared.

If you remain in complete remission for 5 years or more, some doctors may say that you are cured. Still, some cancer cells can remain in your body for many years after treatment. These cells may cause the cancer to come back one day. For cancers that return, most do so within the first 5 years after treatment. But there is a chance that cancer will come back later. For this reason, doctors cannot say for sure that you are cured. The most they can say is that there are no signs of cancer at this time.

Because of the chance that cancer can come back, your doctor will monitor you for many years and do tests to look for signs of cancer's return. They will also look for signs of late effects from the cancer treatments you received.

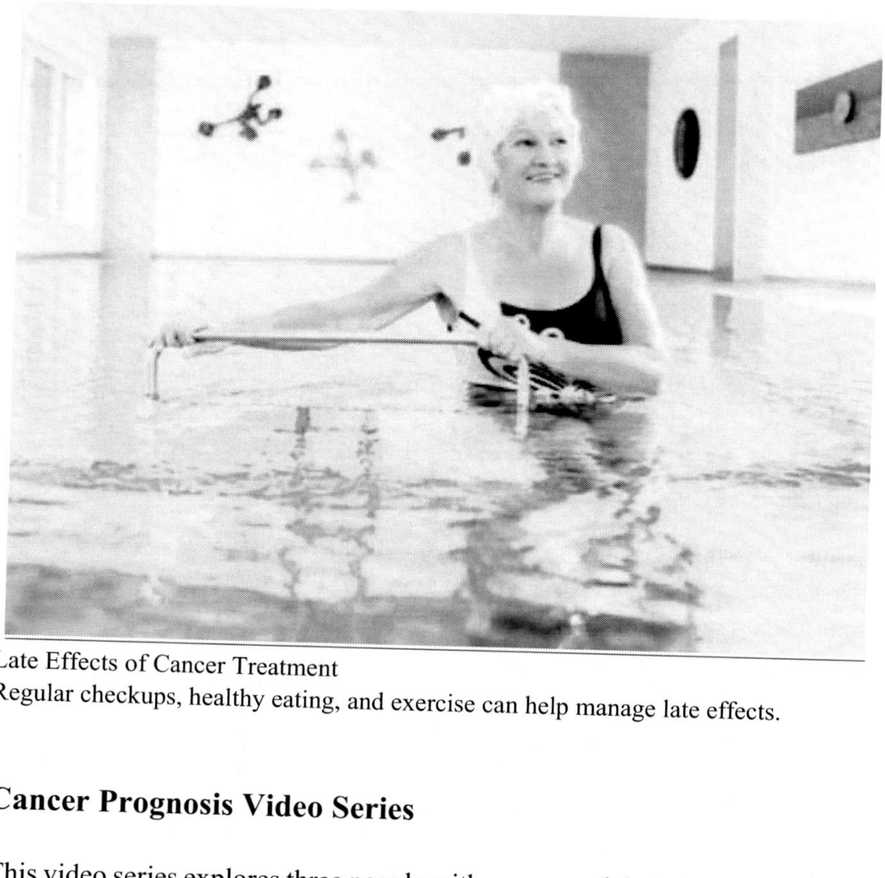

Late Effects of Cancer Treatment
Regular checkups, healthy eating, and exercise can help manage late effects.

Cancer Prognosis Video Series

This video series explores three people with cancer and their doctor's thoughts and feelings about prognosis. The videos explain key points about prognosis and how doctors and patients can talk about it in a clear and supportive way. Two viewer guides are also available: for patients (PDF-210KB) and for provider care teams (PDF-210KB).

Questions to Ask Your Doctor about Your Diagnosis

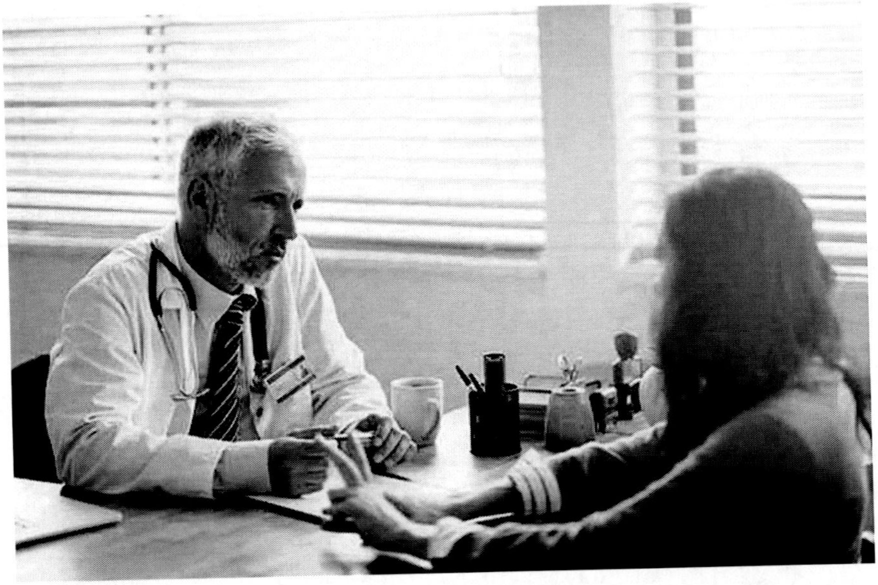

Credit: iStock.

Learning that you have cancer can be a shock and you may feel overwhelmed at first. When you meet with your doctor, you will hear a lot of information. These questions may help you learn more about your cancer and what you can expect next.

- What type of cancer do I have?
- What is the stage of my cancer?
- Has it spread to other areas of my body?
- Will I need more tests before treatment begins? Which ones?
- Which types of doctors do I need to see for my cancer treatment?
- Will you help me find a doctor to give me another opinion on the best treatment plan for me?
- How serious is my cancer?
- What are my chances of survival?

Chapter 4

Cancer Disparities*

National Cancer Institute

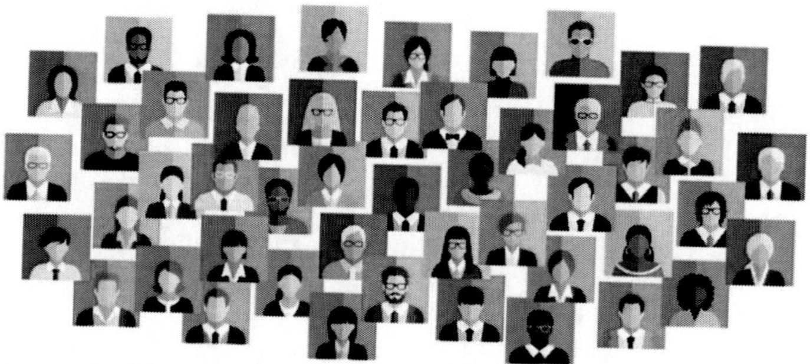

Although cancer incidence and mortality overall are declining in the United States, certain groups continue to be at greater risk of developing or dying from particular cancers.
Credit: iStock

Cancer affects all population groups in the United States, but due to social, environmental, and economic disadvantages, certain groups bear a disproportionate burden of cancer compared with other groups.

Cancer disparities (sometimes called cancer health disparities) are differences in cancer measures such as:

- incidence (new cases)
- prevalence (all existing cases)
- mortality (deaths)
- survival (how long people survive after diagnosis)

---

* This is an edited, reformatted and augmented version of National Cancer Institute Publication.

In: Understanding Cancer
Editor: Angela C. Ray
ISBN: 979-8-89530-769-4

- morbidity (cancer-related health complications)
- survivorship (including quality of life after cancer treatment)
- financial burden of cancer or related health conditions
- screening rates
- stage at diagnosis

Cancer disparities can also be seen when outcomes are improving overall but the improvements are not seen in some groups relative to other groups.

Population groups that may experience cancer disparities include groups defined by race, ethnicity, disability, gender identity, geographic location, income, education, age, sexual orientation, national origin, and other characteristics.

On This Page

Examples of Cancer Disparities

Although cancer incidence and mortality overall are declining in all population groups in the United States, some groups continue to be at increased risk of developing or dying from certain cancers.

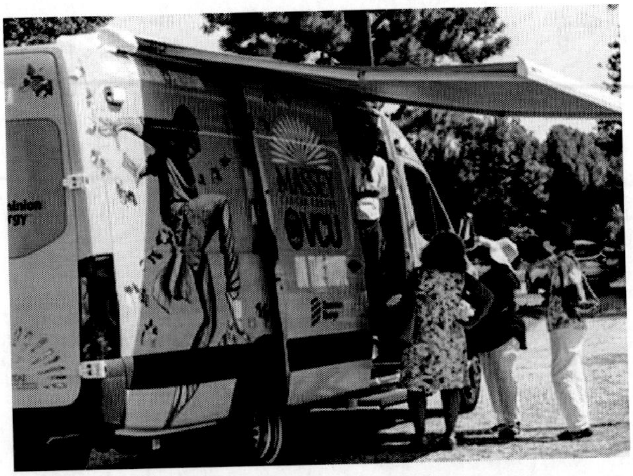

- Putting Cancer Disparities in the Rearview Mirror
- Tackling cancer disparities will require advances and changes that go well beyond the laboratory and doctor's office.

Statistics from NCI's Surveillance, Epidemiology, and End Results Program include information specific to racial and ethnic groups as well as populations defined by age, gender, and geography. Some key cancer incidence and mortality disparities in the United States include:

- Black/African American people have higher death rates than all other racial/ethnic groups for many, although not all, cancer types.
- Despite having slightly lower incidence rates of breast cancer than those of White women, Black/African American women are more likely than White women to die of the disease.
- The incidence rates of colorectal, lung, and cervical cancers are much higher in people who live in rural Appalachia than in those who live in urban areas in the region.
- Although deaths from prostate cancer have dropped substantially in recent decades among all men, Black/African American men are more than twice as likely as White men to die of prostate cancer and continue to have the highest prostate cancer mortality rates among all US racial/ethnic groups.
- People with more education are less likely to die prematurely (before the age of 65) from colorectal cancer than those with less education, regardless of race or ethnicity.
- Hispanic/Latino, Black/African American, and American Indian/Alaska Native women have higher incidence rates of cervical cancer than women of other racial/ethnic groups, with Black/African American women having the highest rates of death from the disease.
- American Indians/Alaska Natives have higher death rates from kidney cancer than any other racial/ethnic group.
- The rates of smoking and alcohol drinking, which increase cancer risk, are higher among lesbian, gay, and bisexual youths than among heterosexual youths.
- American Indians/Alaska Natives have the highest incidence and mortality rates of liver and intrahepatic bile duct cancer, followed by Hispanics/Latinos and Asians/Pacific Islanders.

Contributing Factors

Social Determinants of Health

The Department of Health and Human Services defines social determinants of health as the conditions in the environments where people are born, live, learn, work, play, worship, and age that affect health, functioning, and quality of life.

Cancer disparities reflect the interplay among many factors, including social determinants of health, behavior, biology, and genetics—all of which can have profound effects on health, including cancer risk and outcomes.

Certain groups in the United States experience cancer disparities because they are more likely to encounter obstacles in getting health care.

For example, people with low incomes, low health literacy, or long travel distances to screening or treatment sites, or who lack health insurance, transportation to a medical facility, or paid medical leave are less likely to have recommended cancer screening tests and to be treated according to guidelines than those who don't encounter these obstacles.

People who do not have reliable access to health care are also more likely to be diagnosed with late-stage cancer that might have been treated more effectively if it had been diagnosed at an earlier stage.

Some groups are disproportionately affected by cancer due to environmental conditions. People who live in communities that lack clean water or air may be exposed to cancer-causing substances.

The built environment can also influence behaviors that raise one's risk of cancer. For example, people who live in neighborhoods that lack affordable healthy foods or safe areas for exercise are more likely to have poor diets, be physically inactive, and obese, all of which are risk factors for cancer.

Even people of higher socioeconomic status and those with health insurance may experience cancer disparities. The disparities these individuals experience may reflect the health impact of institutional racism and the chronic stress it causes, conscious or unconscious bias from health providers, mistrust of the health care system, or fatalistic attitudes about cancer.

In some cases, inherited factors or tumor biological factors may, either directly or by interacting with factors such as diet, chronic stress, or tobacco exposure, lead to cancer disparities.

Health Equity

According to the Centers for Disease Control and Prevention, health equity is achieved when every person has the opportunity to attain his or her full health potential and no one is disadvantaged from achieving this potential because of social position or other socially determined circumstances.

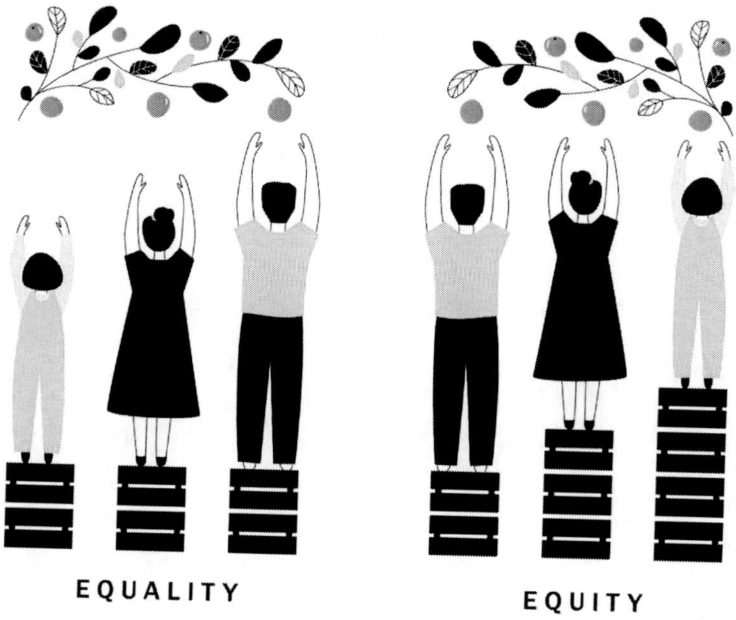

Credit: iStock.

For example, some evidence suggests that there are differences in the genetics, tumor biology, and immune environment of several cancers that arise in Black/African Americans compared with those that arise in people of other racial/ethnic groups. These differences may contribute to disparities in incidence, cancer growth rate, and response to treatment of these cancers.

Cancer disparities may also be exacerbated by the lack of diversity in clinical research participation. Because of this lack of diversity, research results may not be applicable to all populations.

Because many different factors can influence cancer disparities, addressing them is not simple or straightforward. Reducing or eliminating some cancer disparities in the pursuit of health equity will require policy changes to overcome systemic social, racial, and institutional inequalities.

NCI-funded researchers are working to identify other ways to improve outcomes for groups disproportionately affected by cancer. Their research efforts range from designing and implementing culturally appropriate health interventions, to improving access to care and connecting underrepresented populations to clinical trials, to examining biological and genetic factors that may explain differences in rates of fast-growing cancers.

Learn about cancer health disparities research and NCI's efforts to end structural racism in biomedical research.

Chapter 5

Cancer Treatment*

National Cancer Institute

There are many types of cancer treatment. The types of treatment that you have will depend on the type of cancer you have and how advanced it is. Some people with cancer will have only one treatment. But most people have a combination of treatments, such as surgery with chemotherapy and/or radiation therapy. You may also have immunotherapy, targeted therapy, or hormone therapy.

Clinical trials might also be an option for you. Clinical trials are research studies that involve people. Understanding what they are and how they work can help you decide if taking part in a trial is a good option for you.

When you need treatment for cancer, you have a lot to learn and think about. It is normal to feel overwhelmed and confused. But, talking with your doctor and learning all you can about all your treatment options, including clinical trials, can help you make a decision you feel good about. Our *Questions to Ask Your Doctor About Treatment* may help.

Types of Cancer Treatment

Reach out to a cancer information specialist for questions about treatments.

There are many types of cancer treatment. The types of treatment that you receive will depend on the type of cancer you have and how advanced it is.

Some people with cancer will have only one treatment. But most people have a combination of treatments, such as surgery with chemotherapy and radiation therapy.

---

* This is an edited, reformatted and augmented version of National Cancer Institute Publication.

In: Understanding Cancer
Editor: Angela C. Ray
ISBN: 979-8-89530-769-4

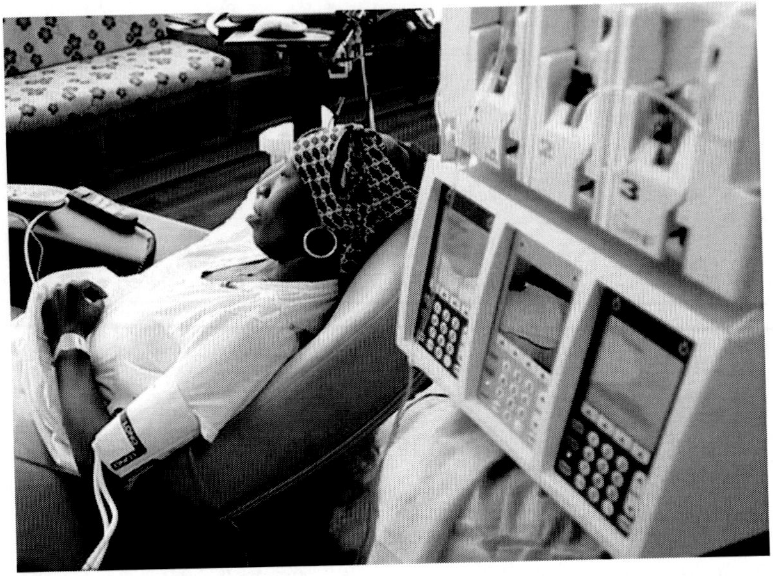

Get Answers >

When you need treatment for cancer, you have a lot to learn and think about. It is normal to feel overwhelmed and confused.

But, talking with your doctor and learning about the types of treatment you may have can help you feel more in control.

Our list of *Questions to Ask Your Doctor About Treatment may help.*

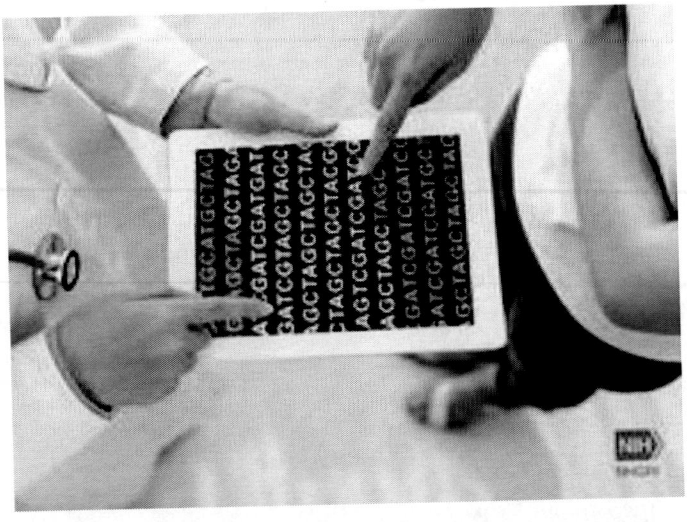

Biomarker Testing for Cancer Treatment

Biomarker testing is a way to look for genes, proteins, and other substances (called biomarkers or tumor markers) that can provide information about cancer. Biomarker testing can help you and your doctor choose a cancer treatment.

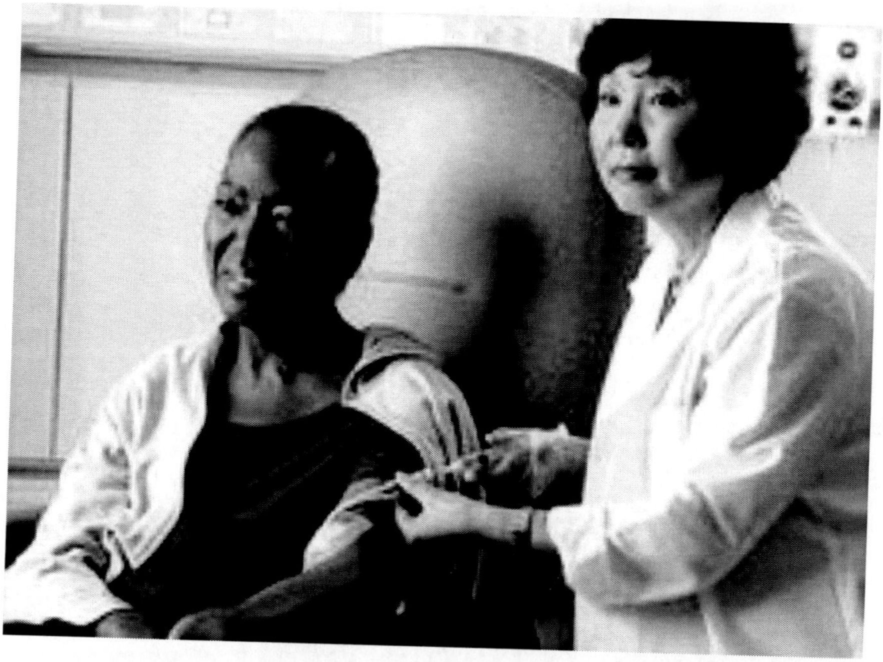

Chemotherapy

Chemotherapy is a type of cancer treatment that uses drugs to kill cancer cells. Learn how chemotherapy works against cancer, why it causes side effects, and how it is used with other cancer treatments.

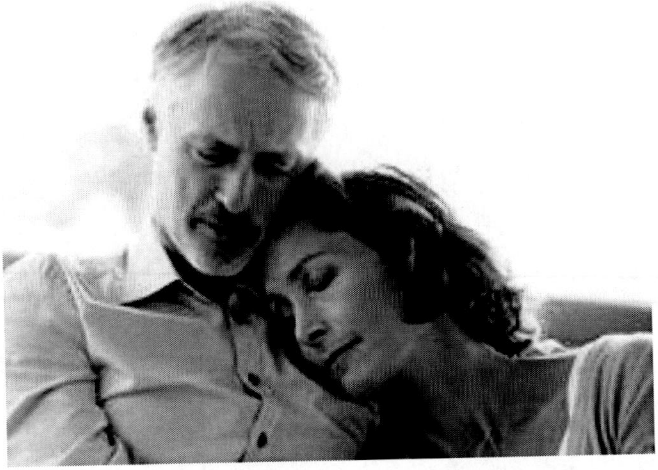

Hormone Therapy

Hormone therapy is a treatment that slows or stops the growth of breast and prostate cancers that use hormones to grow. Learn about the types of hormone therapy and side effects that may happen.

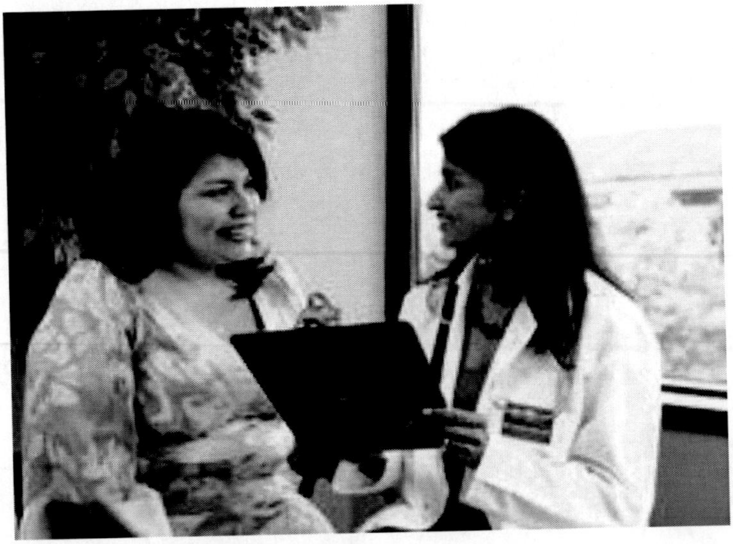

Hyperthermia

Hyperthermia is a type of treatment in which body tissue is heated to as high as 113 °F to help damage and kill cancer cells with little or no harm to normal tissue. Learn about the types of cancer and precancers that hyperthermia is used to treat, how it is given, and the benefits and drawbacks of using hyperthermia.

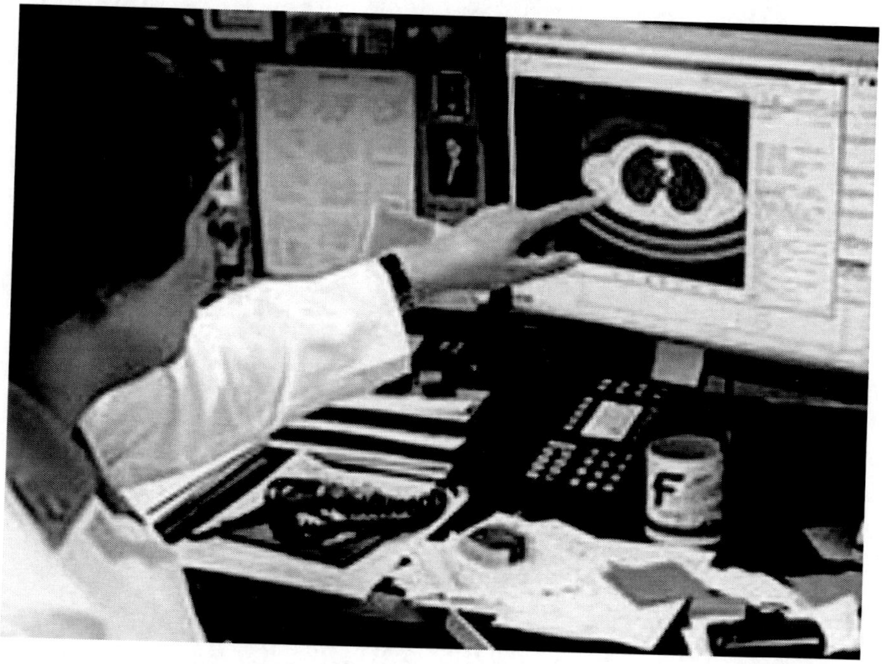

Immunotherapy

Immunotherapy is a type of cancer treatment that helps your immune system fight cancer. This page covers the types of immunotherapy, how it is used against cancer, and what you can expect during treatment.

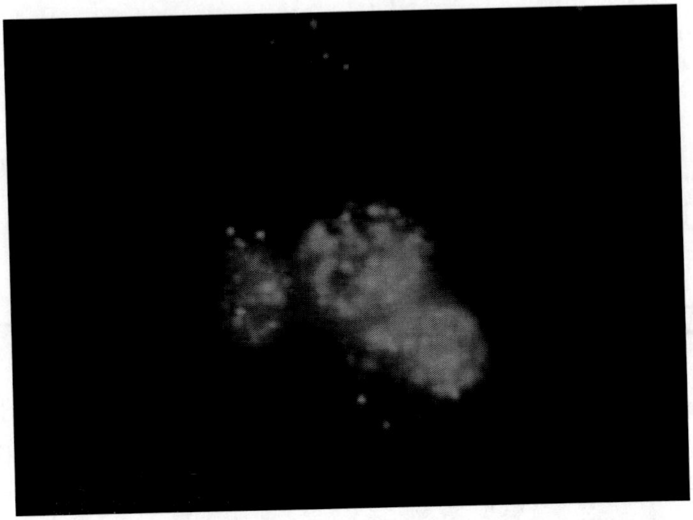

Photodynamic Therapy

Photodynamic therapy uses a drug activated by light to kill cancer and other abnormal cells. Learn how photodynamic therapy works, about the types of cancer and precancers it is used to treat, and the benefits and drawbacks of this treatment.

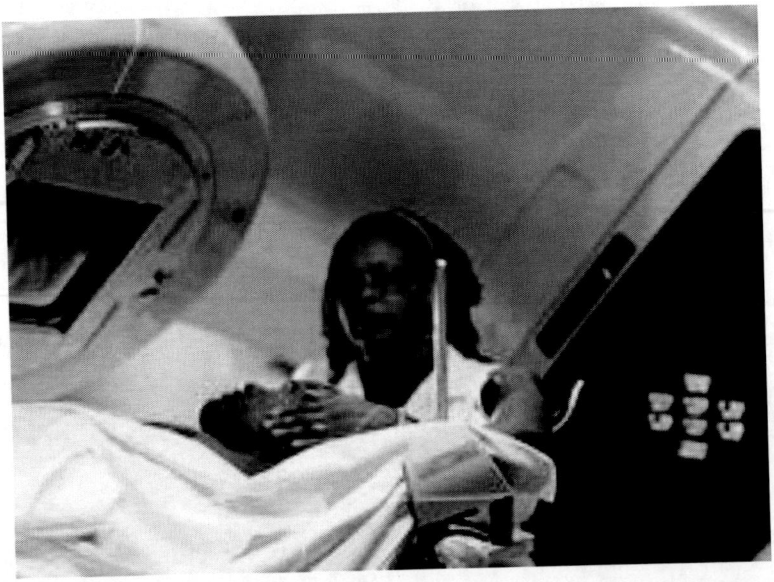

Radiation Therapy

Radiation therapy is a type of cancer treatment that uses high doses of radiation to kill cancer cells and shrink tumors. Learn about the types of radiation, why side effects happen, which side effects you might have, and more.

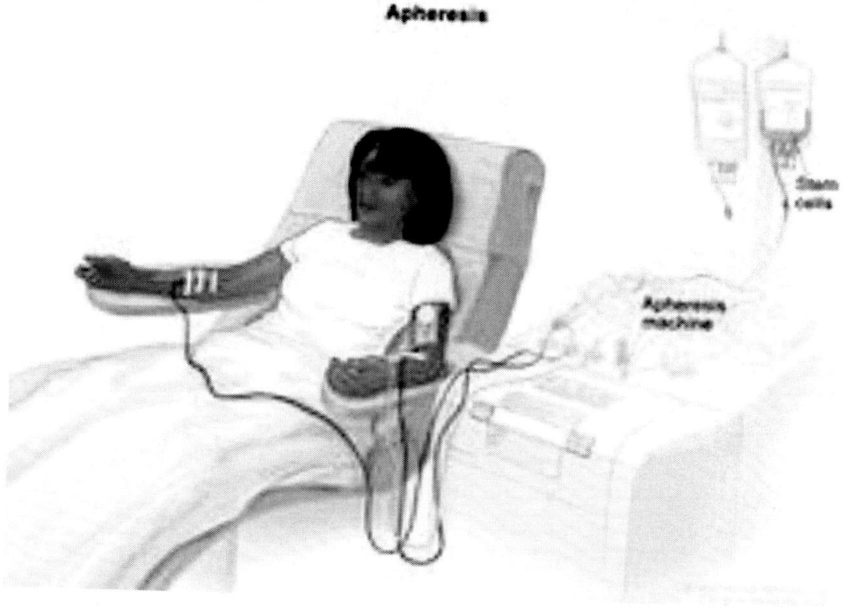

Stem Cell Transplant

Stem cell transplants are procedures that restore stem cells that grow into blood cells in people who have had theirs destroyed by high doses of chemotherapy or radiation therapy. Learn about the types of transplants, side effects that may occur, and how stem cell transplants are used in cancer treatment.

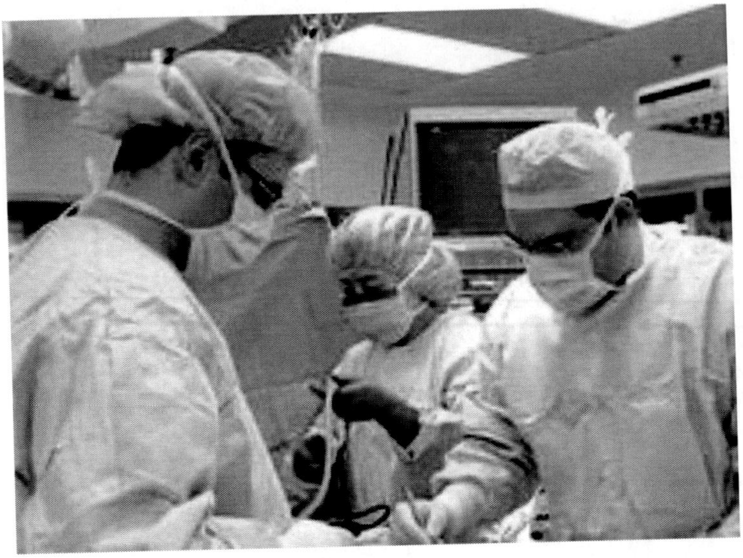

Surgery

When used to treat cancer, surgery is a procedure in which a surgeon removes cancer from your body. Learn the different ways that surgery is used against cancer and what you can expect before, during, and after surgery.

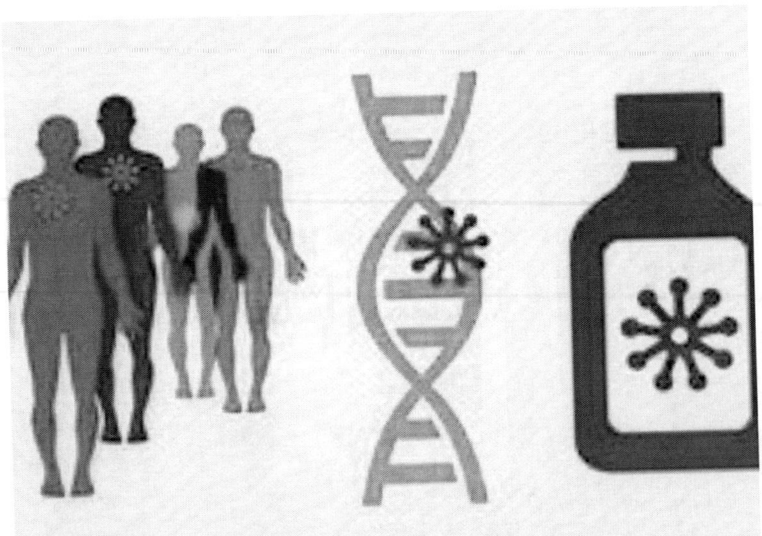

Targeted Therapy

Targeted therapy is a type of cancer treatment that targets the changes in cancer cells that help them grow, divide, and spread. Learn how targeted therapy works against cancer and about common side effects that may occur.

Side Effects of Cancer Treatment

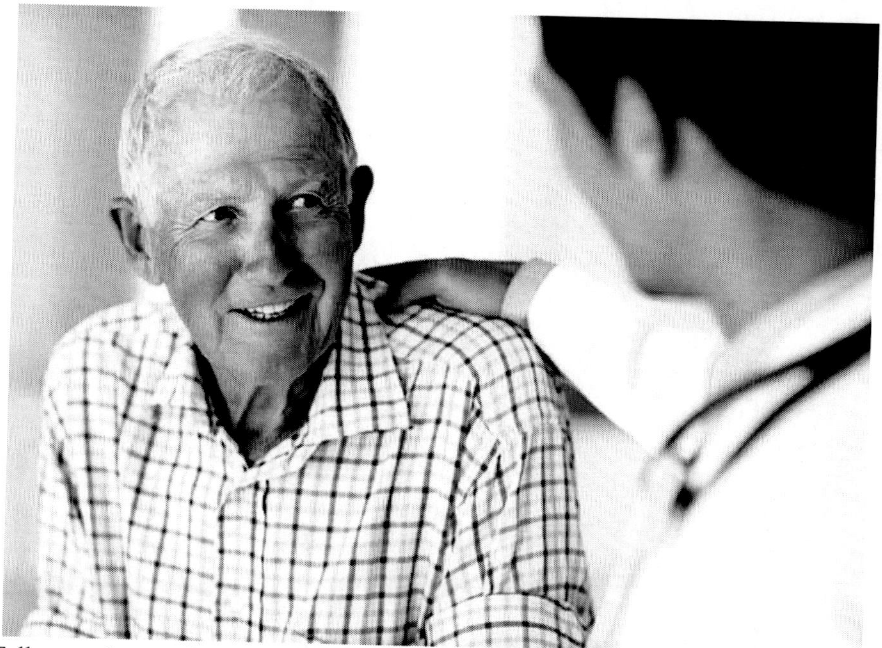

Tell your doctor about side effects you are experiencing, so you get the care and treatment you need to manage these problems.
Credit: iStock.

Cancer treatments and cancer can cause side effects. Side effects are problems that occur when treatment affects healthy tissues or organs. Speak up about any problems you have. Your health care team can treat and/or talk with you about ways to reduce these side effects, so you feel better.

Learn about steps you can take to prevent or manage the side effects listed below:

- Anemia

- Appetite Loss
- Bleeding and Bruising (Thrombocytopenia)
- Bowel Obstruction
- Constipation
- Delirium
- Diarrhea
- Edema (Swelling)
- Fatigue
- Fertility Issues in Boys and Men
- Fertility Issues in Girls and Women
- Flu-Like Symptoms
- Hair Loss (Alopecia)
- Infection and Neutropenia
- Lymphedema
- Memory or Concentration Problems
- Mouth and Throat Problems
- Nausea and Vomiting
- Nerve Problems (Peripheral Neuropathy)
- Organ-Related Inflammation and Immunotherapy
- Pain
- Sexual Health Issues in Men
- Sexual Health Issues in Women
- Skin and Nail Changes
- Sleep Problems
- Urinary and Bladder Problems

Keep in mind that side effects vary from person to person, even among people receiving the same type of cancer treatment.

Complementary and Alternative Medicine

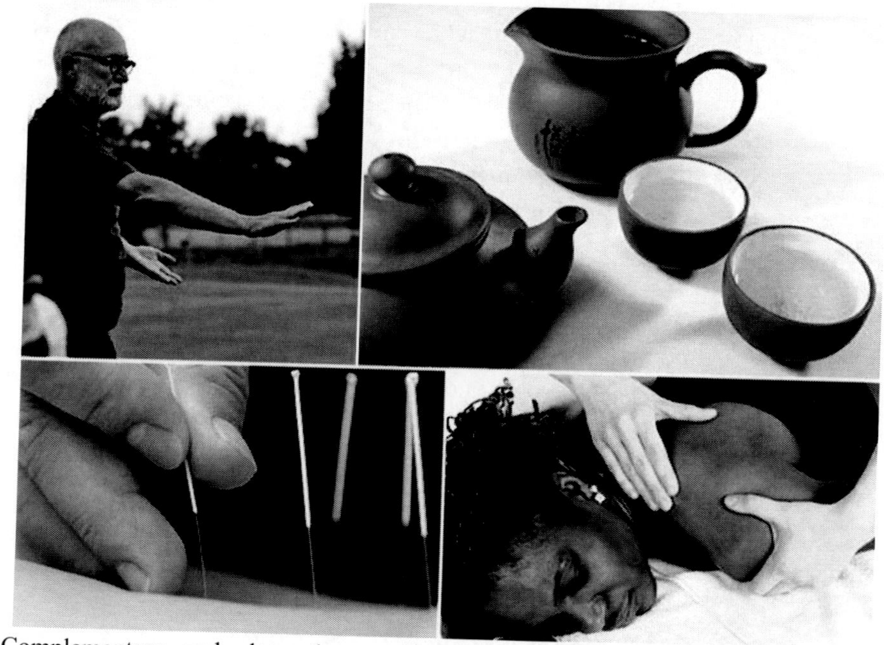

Complementary and alternative medicine includes practices such as massage, acupuncture, tai chi, and drinking green tea.
Credit: iStock.

Complementary and alternative medicine (CAM) is the term for medical products and practices that are not part of standard medical care. People with cancer may use CAM to

- help cope with the side effects of cancer treatments, such as nausea, pain, and fatigue
- comfort themselves and ease the worries of cancer treatment and related stress
- feel that they are doing something to help with their own care
- try to treat or cure their cancer

Integrative medicine is an approach to medical care that combines conventional medicine with CAM practices that have shown through science to be safe and effective. This approach often stresses the patient's preferences, and it attempts to address the mental, physical, and spiritual aspects of health.

Conventional medicine is a system in which health professionals who hold an M.D. (medical doctor) or D.O. (doctor of osteopathy) degree treat symptoms and diseases using drugs, radiation, or surgery. It is also practiced by other health professionals, such as nurses, pharmacists, physician assistants, and therapists. It may also be called *allopathic medicine, biomedicine,* Western, mainstream, or *orthodox medicine*. Some conventional medical care practitioners are also practitioners of CAM.

Standard medical care is treatment that is accepted by medical experts as a proper treatment for a certain type of disease and that is widely used by healthcare professionals. Also called *best practice, standard of care, and standard therapy.*

Complementary medicine is used along with standard medical treatment but is not considered by itself to be standard treatment. One example is using *acupuncture* to help lessen some side effects of cancer treatment. Less research has been done for most types of complementary medicine.

Alternative medicine is used instead of standard medical treatment. One example is using a special diet to treat cancer instead of cancer drugs that are prescribed by an oncologist. Less research has been done for most types of alternative medicine.

Types of Complementary and Alternative Medicine

Scientists learn about CAM therapies every day, but there is still more to learn. This list is meant to be an introduction to what types of CAM are practiced, not an endorsement. Some of the therapies listed below still need more research to prove that they can be helpful. If you have cancer, you should discuss your thoughts about using CAM with your health care provider before using the therapies listed below.

People may use the term "natural," "holistic," "home remedy," or "Eastern Medicine" to refer to CAM. However, experts often use five categories to describe it. These are listed below with examples for each.

Mind–Body Therapies

These combine mental focus, breathing, and body movements to help relax the body and mind. Some examples are

- *meditation:* focused breathing or repetition of words or phrases to quiet the mind and lessen stressful thoughts and feelings.
- *biofeedback:* using special machines, the patient learns how to control certain body functions that are normally out of one's awareness (such as *heart rate* and *blood pressure*).
- *hypnosis:* a trance-like state in which a person becomes more aware and focused on certain feelings, thoughts, images, sensations or behaviors. A person may feel more calm and open to suggestion in order to aid in healing.
- *yoga:* ancient system of practices used to balance the mind and body through stretches and poses, meditation, and controlled breathing
- *tai chi:* a form of gentle exercise and meditation that uses slow sets of body movements and controlled breathing
- *imagery:* focusing on positive images in the mind, such as imagining scenes, pictures, or experiences to help the body heal
- *creative outlets:* interests such as art, music, or dance

Biologically Based Practices

This type of CAM uses things found in nature. Some examples are

- vitamins: nutrients the body needs in small amounts to function and stay healthy
- dietary supplements: products added to the diet that may contain ingredients such as vitamins, minerals, and herbs, to name a few
- botanicals: plants or parts of plants. One type is cannabis.
  - herbs and spices such as turmeric or cinnamon (See Herbs at a Glance)
- special foods or diets

Manipulative And Body-Based Practices

These are based on working with one or more parts of the body. Some examples are

- massage therapy: a therapy where the soft tissues of the body are kneaded, rubbed, tapped, and stroked
- chiropractic therapy: a type of manipulation of the spine, joints, and skeletal system
- reflexology: a type of massage in which pressure is applied to specific points on the feet or hands, which are believed to match up with certain parts of the body

Energy Healing

Energy healing is based on the belief that a vital energy flows through the body. The goal is to balance the energy flow in the patient. There's not enough evidence to support the existence of energy fields. However, there are no harmful effects in using these approaches. Some examples are

- reiki: placing hands lightly on or just above the person with the goal of guiding energy to help a person's own healing response
- therapeutic touch: moving hands over energy fields of the body or gently touching a person's body

Whole Medical Systems

Trial Tests Acupuncture for Pain in Cancer Survivors

Modest pain improvements were seen, although a placebo effect could not be ruled out.

These are healing systems and beliefs that have evolved over time in different cultures and parts of the world. Some examples are

- *Ayurvedic medicine:* a system from India in which the goal is to cleanse the body and restore balance to the body, mind, and spirit. It uses diet, herbal medicines, exercise, meditation, breathing, physical therapy, and other methods.
- *Traditional Chinese medicine:* based on the belief that qi (the body's vital energy) flows along meridians (channels) in the body and keeps a person's spiritual, emotional, mental, and physical health in

balance. It aims to restore the body's balance between two forces called yin and yang.

  - Acupuncture is a common practice in Chinese medicine that involves stimulating certain points on the body to promote health, or to lessen disease symptoms and treatment side effects.

- naturopathic medicine: a system that avoids drugs and surgery. It is based on the use of natural agents such as air, water, light, heat and massage to help the body heal itself. It may also use herbal products, nutrition, acupuncture, and aromatherapy.

For details about specific CAM therapies, NCI provides evidence-based Physician Data Query (PDQ) information for many CAM therapies in versions for both the patient and health professional. Also see the page from the National Center for Complementary and Integrative Health (NCCIH) Cancer and Complementary Health Approaches: What You Need to Know for more details about CAM and some of the current research.

The Safety of CAM

Some CAM therapies have undergone careful evaluation and have been found to be generally safe and effective. These include acupuncture, yoga, and meditation to name a few. However, there are others that do not work, may be harmful, or could interact negatively with your medicines.

Natural Does Not Mean Safe

CAM therapies include a wide variety of botanicals and nutritional products, such as herbal and dietary supplements, and vitamins. These products do not have to be approved by the Food and Drug Administration (FDA) before being sold to the public. Also, a prescription isn't needed to buy them. Therefore, it's up to you to decide what's best for you. Some tips to keep in mind are below.

- Herbal supplements may be harmful when taken by themselves, with other substances, or in large doses. For example, some studies have shown that kava kava, an herb that has been used to help with stress and anxiety, may cause liver damage. And St. John, which some people use for depression, may cause certain cancer drugs to not work as well as they should.

- Tell your doctor if you're taking any dietary supplements, even vitamins, no matter how safe you think they are. This is very important. Even though there may be ads or claims that something has been used for years, they do not prove that it's safe or effective. This is even more true when combined with your medicines.

Diet Alone Cannot Control Cancer

It's common for people with cancer to have questions about different foods to eat during treatment. Yet it's important to know there isn't just one food or special diet that has proved to control cancer.

- We all have different bodies and ways we metabolize food. What is best for someone else may not be right for you. Because of your individual nutrition needs, it's best to talk with the doctor in charge of your treatment about the foods you should be eating.
- It's always important for you to have a healthy diet, but especially now. Do the best you can to have a well-rounded approach, eating a variety of foods that are good for you. For advice about eating during and after cancer treatment, see the NCI booklet, Eating Hints.

It's important to know that there are no studies that prove that any special diet, food, vitamin, mineral, dietary supplement, herb, or combination of these can slow cancer, cure it, or keep it from coming back. In fact, some of these products can cause other problems by changing how your cancer treatment works.

Talk With Your Doctor Before You Use CAM

Cancer patients who want to use CAM should talk with their doctor or nurse. This is an important step because things that seem safe could be harmful or even interfere with your cancer treatment. It's also a good idea to learn if the therapy you're thinking about has been proven to do what it claims to do. Some examples of questions to ask:

What types of CAM therapies might help me

- reduce my stress and anxiety?
- feel less tired?
- deal with cancer symptoms and side effects, such as pain or nausea?
- sleep better?

Always tell your doctor about what complementary health approaches you're using. Whether it's something that seems simple, such as massage or a type of exercise, it's good to let your doctor or nurse know what you're doing. Don't forget to tell them about over-the-counter and prescription medicines that you're taking. Make a list in advance and take it with you.

Don't be afraid to ask questions. It's okay to feel hesitant when asking about using CAM. But doctors want to know what concerns you have so they can give you the best possible care. Let them know that you would like to use CAM methods and want their input.

Questions to Ask a CAM Practitioner

Choosing a CAM practitioner should be done with the same care as choosing a doctor. Ask your doctor, nurse, or social worker at your cancer center to help you find a practitioner for you. For more tips to help you in your search, see 6 Things to Know When Selecting a Complementary Health Practitioner from NCCIH. Once you choose someone to see, questions you may want to ask include:

- What types of CAM do you practice?
- What are your training and qualifications?
- Do you see other patients with my type of cancer?
- Will you work with my doctor if necessary?

Questions to Ask About the CAM Therapy

- How can this help me?

- Do you know of studies that prove it helps?
- What are the risks and side effects?
- Will this interfere with my cancer treatment?
- How long will I be on the therapy?
- What will it cost? Do you take insurance?
- Do you have information that I can read about it?

Questions to Ask Yourself About the CAM Practitioner

- Do I feel comfortable with this person?
- Do I like how the office looks and feels?
- Do I like the staff?
- Does this person support standard cancer treatments?
- How far am I willing to travel for treatment?
- Is it easy to get an appointment?
- Are the office hours good for me?
- Will insurance cover my costs? (Call your health plan or insurer to see whether they cover CAM therapies. Many are not covered.)

Clinical Trials to Test CAM Therapies

NCI and the National Center for Complementary and Integrative Health (NCCIH) are currently sponsoring or cosponsoring clinical trials that test CAM treatments and therapies in people. Some study the effects of complementary approaches used in addition to conventional treatments, and some compare alternative therapies with conventional treatments. You can find a list of all cancer CAM clinical trials here.

Dr. Jeffrey D. White, OCCAM Director, explains the use of complementary and alternative medicine in cancer.

Patients, their families, and their health care providers can learn about CAM therapies and practitioners from the following government agencies:

- National Center for Complementary and Integrative Health
- NCI Office of Cancer Complementary and Alternative Medicine
- NIH Office of Dietary Supplements

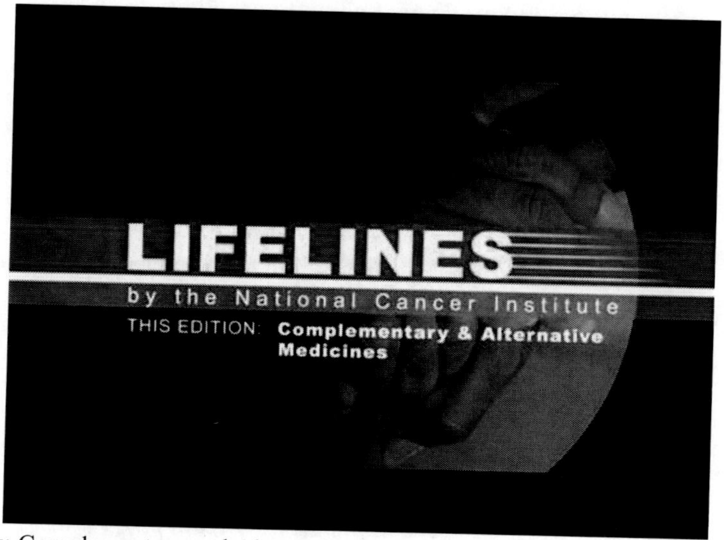

Lifelines: Complementary and Alternative Medicine.

Questions to Ask Your Doctor about Treatment

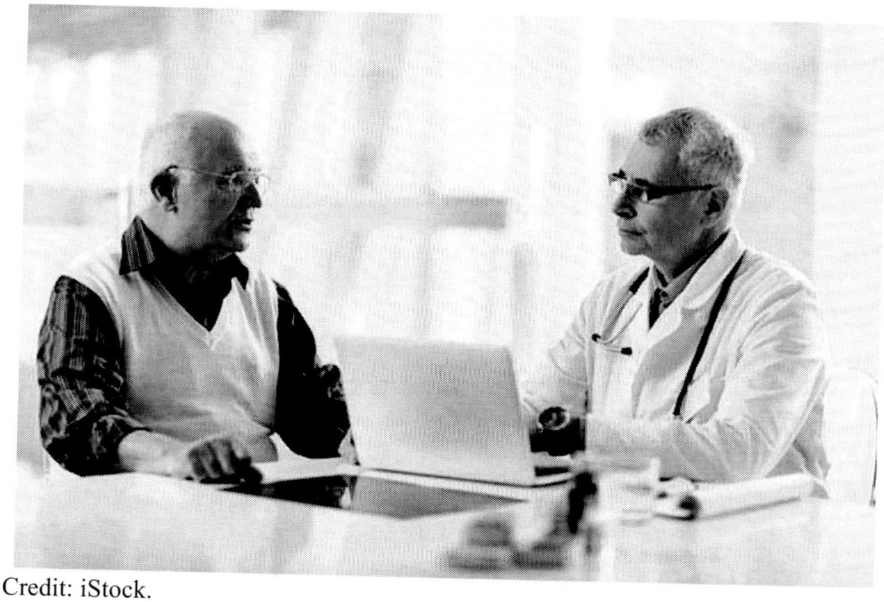

Credit: iStock.

You may want to ask your doctor some of the following questions before you decide on your cancer treatment.

Questions about Cancer Treatment

- What are treatments for my type and stage of cancer?
- Where can I find more information about the types of cancer treatments?
- What are the benefits and risks of each of these treatments?
- What treatment do you recommend? Why do you think it is best for me?
- When will I need to start treatment?
- Will I need to be in the hospital for treatment? If so, for how long?
- What is my chance of recovery with this treatment?
- How will we know if the treatment is working?
- Would a clinical trial (research study) be right for me?
- How do I find out about studies for my type and stage of cancer?

Questions About Finding a Specialist and Getting a Second Opinion

- Will I need a specialist(s) for my cancer treatment?
- Will you help me find a doctor for a second opinion on the best treatment plan for me?

Questions about What Happens during Treatment

- Where will I go for treatment?
- How is the treatment given?
- How long will each treatment session take?
- How many treatment sessions will I have?
- Should a family member or friend come with me to my treatment sessions?

- How will I feel after each treatment? Will I be able to go about my day or should I plan to rest?
- Will I be able to work? Should I think about going part-time?
- Will treatment affect my appetite or make it hard to eat?

Questions about Side Effects

- What are the possible *side effects* of the treatment?
- What side effects may happen during or between my treatment sessions?
- Are there any side effects that I should call you about right away?
- Are there any lasting side effects of the treatment?
- Will this treatment affect my ability to have children?
- Will treatment affect my appetite or make it hard to eat?
- How can I prevent or treat side effects?

Questions About Medicines and Other Products You Might Be Taking

- Do I need to tell you about the medicines I am taking now?
- Should I tell you about dietary supplements (such as vitamins, minerals, herbs, or fish oil) that I am taking?
- Could any drugs or supplements change the way that cancer treatment works?

Chapter 6

Cancer Statistics*

National Cancer Institute

Cancer has a major impact on society in the United States and across the world. Cancer statistics describe what happens in large groups of people and provide a picture in time of the burden of cancer on society.

Statistics tell us things such as how many people are diagnosed with and die from cancer each year, the number of people who are currently living after a cancer diagnosis, the average age at diagnosis, and the numbers of people who are still alive at a given time after diagnosis. They also tell us about differences among groups defined by age, sex, racial/ethnic group, geographic location, and other categories.

Cancer statistics also help us see trends. By looking at cancer rates over time, we can track changes in the risk of developing and dying from specific cancers as well as cancer overall.

For information about chances of surviving cancer and prognosis, see Understanding Cancer Prognosis. NCI also has a collection of statistical summaries for a number of common cancer types.

Although statistical trends are usually not directly applicable to individual patients, they are essential for governments, policy makers, health professionals, and researchers to understand the impact of cancer on the population and to develop strategies to address the challenges that cancer poses to the society at large. Statistical trends are also important for measuring the success of efforts to control and manage cancer.

---

* This is an edited, reformatted and augmented version of National Cancer Institute Publication.

In: Understanding Cancer
Editor: Angela C. Ray
ISBN: 979-8-89530-769-4

Statistics at a Glance: The Burden of Cancer in the United States

- In 2024, an estimated 2,001,140 new cases of cancer will be diagnosed in the United States and 611,720 people will die from the disease.
- The most common cancers (listed in descending order according to estimated new cases in 2024) are breast cancer, prostate cancer, lung and bronchus cancer, colon and rectum cancer, melanoma of the skin, bladder cancer, kidney and renal pelvis cancer, non-Hodgkin lymphoma, endometrial cancer, pancreatic cancer, leukemia, thyroid cancer, and liver cancer.
- Prostate, lung, and colorectal cancers account for an estimated 48% of all cancers diagnosed in men in 2024. For women, the three most common cancers are breast, lung, and colorectal, and they will account for an estimated 51% of all new cancer diagnoses in women in 2024.
- The rate of new cases of cancer (cancer incidence) is 440.5 per 100,000 men and women per year (based on 2017–2021 cases).
- The cancer death rate (cancer mortality) is 146.0 per 100,000 men and women per year (based on 2018–2022 deaths).
- The cancer mortality rate is higher among men than women (173.2 per 100,000 men and 126.4 per 100,000 women). When comparing groups based on race/ethnicity and sex, cancer mortality is highest in non-Hispanic Black men (208.3 per 100,000) and lowest in non-Hispanic Asian/Pacific Islander women (82.6 per 100,000).
- As of January 2022, there were an estimated 18.1 million cancer survivors in the United States. The number of cancer survivors is projected to increase to 22.5 million by 2032.
- Approximately 40.5% of men and women will be diagnosed with cancer at some point during their lifetimes (based on 2017–2019 data).
- In 2024, an estimated 14,910 children and adolescents ages 0 to 19 will be diagnosed with cancer and 1,590 will die of the disease.
- Estimated national expenditures for cancer care in the United States in 2020 were $208.9 billion. In future years, costs are likely to increase as the population ages and more people have cancer. Costs

are also likely to increase as new, and often more expensive, treatments are adopted as standards of care.

Statistics at a Glance: The Burden of Cancer Worldwide

- Cancer is among the leading causes of death worldwide. In 2022, there were almost 20 million new cases and 9.7 million cancer-related deaths worldwide.
- By 2040, the number of new cancer cases per year is expected to rise to 29.9 million and the number of cancer-related deaths to 15.3 million.
- Generally, cancer rates are highest in countries whose populations have the highest life expectancy, education level, and standard of living. But for some cancer types, such as cervical cancer, the reverse is true, and the incidence rate is highest in countries in which the population ranks low on these measures.

Source: International Agency for Research on CancerExit Disclaimer

U.S. Cancer Mortality Trends

The best indicator of progress against cancer is a change in age-adjusted mortality (death) rates, although other measures, such as quality of life, are also important. Incidence is also important, but it is not always straightforward to interpret changes in incidence. A rise in incidence can reflect a real increase in disease occurrence, such as when an increase in exposure to a risk factor causes more cases of cancer. In such a scenario the increased incidence would likely lead to a rise in deaths from the cancer. On the other hand, the incidence of cancer may rise due to a new screening test that detects many cancer cases that would not have caused a problem during someone's life (called overdiagnosis). In this example, the incidence of the cancer would increase, but death rates would not change.

Mortality trends, when compared with incidence trends, can also provide evidence of improved treatments. If death rates drop faster than incidence (or if death rates drop while incidence is rising), this may reflect the availability of better treatments. For example, statistical evidence suggests that improved treatments have likely made a substantial contribution to recent sharp declines in the lung cancer mortality rate.

In the United States, the overall cancer death rate has declined since the early 1990s. Part 1 of the most recent Annual Report to the Nation on the Status of Cancer, released in October 2022, shows that overall cancer death rates decreased by:

- 2.3% per year among men from 2015 to 2019
- 1.9% per year among women from 2015 to 2019
- 1.5% per year among children ages 0–14 from 2015 to 2019

Although death rates for many individual cancer types have also declined, rates for a few cancers have not changed or even increased.

As the overall cancer death rate has declined, the number of cancer survivors has increased. These trends show that progress is being made against the disease, but much work remains. Although rates of smoking, a major cause of cancer, have declined, the rates of other risk factors, such as obesity, have increased in the United States. Also, the U.S. population is aging, and cancer rates increase with age.

The Surveillance, Epidemiology, and End Results (SEER) Program

NCI's Surveillance, Epidemiology, and End Results (SEER) Program collects and publishes cancer incidence and survival data from population-based cancer registries that cover approximately 48% of the U.S. population. The SEER program website has more detailed cancer statistics, including population statistics for common types of cancer, customizable graphs and tables, and interactive tools.

The Annual Report to the Nation on the Status of Cancer provides an annual update of cancer incidence, mortality, and trends in the United States. This report is jointly authored by experts from NCI, the Centers for Disease Control and Prevention, American Cancer Society, and the North American Association of Central Cancer Registries.

Part 1 of the most recent report included a special section about trends in pancreatic cancer. Part 2, released in September 2023, focused on the effect of the COVID-19 pandemic on new cases and deaths from certain cancers. For example, new diagnoses of six major cancer types fell sharply from March to May of 2020, at the start of the pandemic. By July 2020, diagnoses of all of these cancer types except one (prostate cancer) had returned to pre-pandemic levels.

Chapter 7

Cancer Clinical Trials: Federal Actions and Selected Non-Federal Practices to Facilitate Diversity of Patients*

United States Government Accountability Office

Abbreviations

CDMRP	Congressionally Directed Medical Research Programs
CMS	Centers for Medicare & Medicaid Services
DOD	Department of Defense
FDA	Food and Drug Administration
HHS	Department of Health and Human Services
NCI	National Cancer Institute
NIH	National Institutes of Health
VA	Department of Veterans Affairs

Why GAO Did This Study

Diverse representation in clinical trials is important to ensure the safety and efficacy of treatments for the patient population likely to use the treatment being studied. It is also important from an equity perspective as these trials often represent the best available health care. Despite more than 3 decades of

* This is an edited, reformatted and augmented version of the United States Government Accountability Office Report to Congressional Committees, Publication No. GAO-23-105245, dated December 2022.

In: Understanding Cancer
Editor: Angela C. Ray
ISBN: 979-8-89530-769-4

government policies intended to improve clinical trial diversity, certain groups remain consistently underrepresented in cancer clinical trials. Those groups include certain racial and ethnic groups, adolescents and young adults, older adults, women, low-income individuals, and individuals from rural communities.

The Henrietta Lacks Enhancing Cancer Research Act of 2019 and House Appropriations Report 116-450 each included a provision that GAO study diverse representation of patients in cancer clinical trials. This report describes (1) actions federal agencies have taken to facilitate enrollment of patients from diverse backgrounds in cancer clinical trials and (2) practices used by selected non-federal cancer centers to facilitate enrollment of patients from diverse backgrounds in cancer clinical trials.

GAO interviewed officials and reviewed documents from federal agencies that fund or conduct cancer clinical trials.

GAO also identified 17 cancer centers with a history of enrolling diverse populations in cancer clinical trials and asked them to describe relevant practices that facilitated such enrollment. GAO identified practices facilitating diverse enrollment that were described by or about these centers.

What GAO Found

GAO found that both federal agencies and selected non-federal cancer centers took actions to facilitate participation of patients from diverse backgrounds in cancer clinical trials. Generally, these actions addressed a variety of barriers to participation that are often cited in the literature.

The Department of Health and Human Services, Department of Defense, and Department of Veterans Affairs took actions that have the goal of increasing the proportion of patients from diverse backgrounds enrolled in federally funded cancer clinical trials. These efforts are focused on developing research collaborations, modifying research practices, reducing barriers to patient participation, and collecting and sharing data.

Federal Actions to Facilitate Diversity in Cancer Clinical Trials

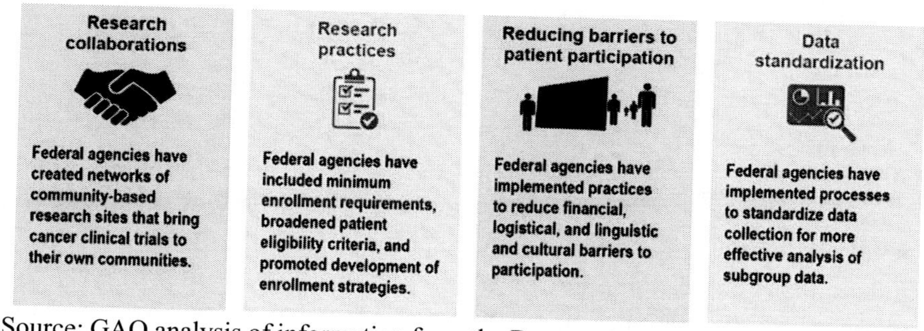

Source: GAO analysis of information from the Department of Defense, Department of Health and Human Services, and Department of Veterans Affairs. | GAO-23-105245.

The 17 non-federal cancer centers in GAO's review implemented practices to facilitate the enrollment of patients from diverse backgrounds that were focused on four areas: organization, community, workforce, and patients. Fifteen of the centers implemented practices in at least three of these four areas.

Selected Cancer Center Practices to Facilitate Diversity in Cancer Clinical Trials

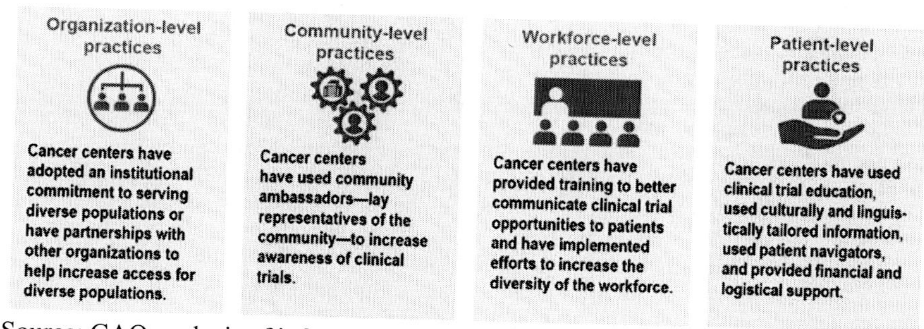

Source: GAO analysis of information about the 17 selected cancer centers. | GAO-23-105245.

December 19, 2022

Congressional Committees

Diverse patient representation in clinical trials is important to ensure the safety and efficacy of treatments for the population likely to use the treatment being studied.[1] Ideally, these trials analyze differences in the safety or efficacy of a treatment amongst different groups to identify biological and social factors that may affect health. For some drugs, these differences have resulted in population-specific information in labeling about dosage or warnings.[2] In addition, diverse representation among patients in clinical trials is important to ensure equity, such that all individuals have access to clinical research, which in many settings, represents the best available health care.[3]

The federal government has made increasing diversity in clinical trials a policy focus for more than 3 decades, yet numerous groups remain underrepresented. For example, the National Institutes of Health (NIH) was mandated to include women and persons from racial and ethnic groups other than non-Hispanic White populations in clinical trials.[4] However, an analysis that searched NIH's clinical trials data base in January 2013 found that NIH's National Cancer Institute (NCI) sponsored or co-sponsored 10,000 clinical trials, and that less than 2 percent of these trials focused on racial or ethnic groups other than non-Hispanic White.[5] Further, a study that examined all

---

[1] The National Institutes of Health (NIH) defines a clinical trial as a research study in which one or more human subjects are prospectively assigned to one or more interventions that may include placebo or other control) to evaluate the effects of those interventions on health-related biomedical or behavioral outcomes. In other words, patients or participants are assigned to a treatment option (which may include one that is actually no treatment, such as with a pill that has no medical component. NCI notes that its definition of clinical trials includes trials to test new methods of screening, prevention, diagnosis, or treatment.

[2] See B. E. Bierer et al., *Achieving Diversity, Inclusion, and Equity in Clinical Research: Guidance Document Version 1.1* (Cambridge and Boston, MA: Multi-Regional Clinical Trials (MRCT) Center of Brigham and Women's Hospital and Harvard, 2021). accessed July 6,2021 https://mrctcenter.org/diversity-in-clinical-trials/.

[3] National Academies of Sciences, Engineering, and Medicine, *Improving Representation in Clinical Trials and Research: Building Research Equity for Women and Underrepresented Groups* (Washington, DC: The National Academies Press, 2022) accessed May 17, 2022, https://doi.org/10.17226/26479.

[4] National Institutes of Health Revitalization Act of 1993, Pub. L. No. 103-43, § 131, 107 Stat. 122, 133-35.

[5] The review notes that other trials may have included patients from a variety of racial and ethnic groups, but such groups were not the primary focus. M. S. Chen et al., "Twenty Years Post-NIH Revitalization Act: Renewing the Case for Enhancing Minority Participation in Cancer Clinical Trials," *Cancer,* vol. 120, no. 7 (2014).

cancer drug approvals granted by the Food and Drug Administration (FDA) from July 2008 through June 2018 found that Black and Hispanic patients in the U.S. were consistently underrepresented in the clinical trials supporting those drug applications when compared to the proportion of cancer incidence and mortality among Blacks and Hispanics in the U.S.[6] Other groups, such as adolescents and young adults, older adults, women, low-income individuals, and individuals from rural communities have also been underrepresented in cancer clinical trials.

The Henrietta Lacks Enhancing Cancer Research Act of 2019 and House Appropriations Report 116-450 each included a provision that we study the diverse representation of patients in cancer clinical trials.[7] This report describes

1. actions federal agencies have taken to facilitate enrollment of patients from diverse backgrounds in cancer clinical trials and
2. practices used by selected cancer centers to facilitate enrollment of patients from diverse backgrounds in cancer clinical trials.

In this report, we focused on groups of patients from diverse backgrounds in terms of racial and ethnic groups, adolescents and young adults, older adults, women, low-income individuals, and individuals from rural communities because they were either specified in the legislation or had been cited in scientific literature as underrepresented groups in clinical trials.

To describe actions federal agencies have taken to facilitate enrollment of patients from diverse backgrounds in cancer clinical trials, we interviewed officials from federal agencies that fund or conduct cancer clinical trials, and develop and maintain policies related to such trials. Specifically, we interviewed officials from agencies within the Department of Health and Human Services (HHS)—including NIH, FDA, and the Centers for Medicare & Medicaid Services (CMS)—the Department of Veterans Affairs (VA), and the Department of Defense (DOD). We also reviewed and analyzed

---

[6] J. M. Loree et al., "Disparity of Race Reporting and Representation in Clinical Trials Leading to Cancer Drug Approvals from 2008 to 2018." *JAMA Oncology*, vol. 5, no. 10 (2019).

[7] Pub. L. No. 116-291, § 3, 134 Stat. 4894, 4895 (2021); H.R. Rep. No. 116-450, at 93 (2020). The Henrietta Lacks Enhancing Cancer Research Act of 2019 includes Congressional finding that scientists used tumor cells from Henrietta Lacks for more than 20 years, without her or her family's consent. The cells have contributed to many scientific advances such as the development of the polio vaccine and other drug treatments.

documents from these agencies outlining relevant policies, procedures, and programs related to clinical trial participation.

To describe practices used by selected cancer centers to facilitate enrollment of patients from diverse backgrounds in cancer clinical trials, we first identified non-federal cancer centers that have been effective at enrolling such patients or recognized in published literature for enrolling diverse populations in cancer trials.[8] To do so, we conducted a literature search and interviewed stakeholders. We used the literature search to identify articles demonstrating the ability to enroll patients from diverse groups in cancer clinical trials, or review articles that recognized such centers. We also asked stakeholders to identify cancer centers that have been effective in enrolling patients from diverse backgrounds in cancer clinical trials or articles that might provide such information. Based on this, we identified 17 cancer centers that met our selection criteria and focused on cancer clinical trials. We use the word "centers" to describe these cancer centers and institutes.[9] We asked officials from the 17 selected centers to identify relevant practices that facilitate enrollment of patients from diverse backgrounds in cancer clinical trials through a questionnaire we provided. We did not independently verify the information reported by the centers in their response to the questionnaires we sent them. We also reviewed documents provided by the centers and published literature about the centers.

To address both objectives, we also conducted interviews with a range of stakeholders who could provide a variety of perspectives on issues related to diversity in cancer clinical trials, actions taken by the federal government, and practices for facilitating enrollment of diverse groups of patients in cancer clinical trials. Specifically, we interviewed representatives from four organizations that represent a variety of perspectives in patient advocacy, six that represent clinical research, and three that represent the pharmaceutical industry. We identified these stakeholders through our review of literature and these interviews. The information we obtained from these interviews with stakeholders is not generalizable; however, it provides insight into issues related to diversity in cancer clinical trials. (A detailed description of our scope and methodology is in app. I.)

---

[8] For the purposes of this report, cancer centers are health care organizations and groups of health care organizations that provide care for people with cancer and conduct cancer clinical trials.

[9] The centers we identified for this report do not constitute all cancer centers that have had increased enrollment of diverse populations into cancer clinical trials.

We conducted this performance audit from May 2021 to December 2022 in accordance with generally accepted government auditing standards. Those standards require that we plan and perform the audit to obtain sufficient, appropriate evidence to provide a reasonable basis for our findings and conclusions based on our audit objectives. We believe that the evidence obtained provides a reasonable basis for our findings and conclusions based on our audit objectives.

Background

Clinical Trials

Clinical trials are studies to test new drugs, already approved drugs, devices, or other forms of treatment, prevention, or supportive care. Clinical trials provide data about the safety and effectiveness of medical products and health care interventions. Funders of clinical trials are also referred to as clinical trial sponsors. Generally, trial sponsors evaluate the design of a clinical trial, often using a technical review process such as peer review, and with require the approval of an Institutional Review Board.[10]

Clinical trial settings. Clinical trials can take place in a variety of settings (e.g., academic hospitals, community hospitals, and specialty treatment centers) and geographic locations. Some clinical trials may be led by a particular research institution, such as a cancer center, but also have multiple community sites that enroll and treat patients in the trial.

Clinical trial funding. Most clinical trials that lead to drug approvals are funded by pharmaceutical companies, and most participants in cancer clinical trials are enrolled outside of the U. S. For example, one study found that of the trials funded in 2014, the number of clinical trials funded by the pharmaceutical industry was more than 6 times greater than the number funded by NIH.[11] In the case of cancer clinical trials, those not funded by pharmaceutical companies are typically funded by federal agencies, academic institutions, and other organizations. The American Cancer Society Cancer Action Network reported that the trials funded by NCI tend to compare one

[10] Institutional Review Boards are formal groups that review and monitor research involving human participants. The groups have the power to approve, require modifications to, or disapprove research. The groups serve to protect the rights and welfare of the participants.

[11] S. Ehrhardt, L. J. Appel, and C. L. Meinert, "Trends in National Institutes of Health Funding for Clinical Trials Registered in ClincialTrials.gov," *JAMA,* vol. 314, no. 23 (2015).

treatment approach against another, whereas those funded by pharmaceutical companies are designed to receive FDA approval for either new drugs or new uses of an already approved drug.[12] FDA has reported that for clinical trials used to support new drugs from 2015 through 2019, 65 percent of clinical trial participants are enrolled in trial settings outside of the U.S.[13]

Clinical trial staff. Clinical trials are led by a principal investigator who is typically a physician. We refer to these principal investigators as "researchers" in this report. These researchers generally have control over the details of the trial, including how participants are recruited and enrolled into the trial, and the data that the trial will gather. They also are responsible for providing oversight of the trial to ensure it is conducted in accordance with the plans. The clinical trial staff may include staff such as research nurses who educate patients about a trial; doctoral-level researchers—such as statisticians and population scientists—who provide expertise in developing the trial structure; staff who manage the collection of data throughout the trial; and physicians, nurses, and other health care providers who provide medical care to clinical trial patients as needed.

Clinical trial participants. Clinical trial participants are those people who enroll in a clinical trial. They may be people with a particular disease or they may be healthy volunteers. Participants may learn about trials from their doctor or from online clinical trial databases. They must meet certain eligibility criteria set by the trial to participate; these criteria can include characteristics such as age, sex, the type and stage of their disease, their previous medical treatment, and other medical conditions. For purposes of this report, we refer to clinical trial participants as "patients."

Federal Agencies That Fund and Conduct Cancer Trials

Federally funded cancer clinical trials are primarily funded by HHS agencies such as NIH, and within NIH, specifically NCI. Other agencies that fund or conduct cancer trials include DOD, through the Congressionally Directed Medical Research Programs (CDMRP) and the John P. Murtha Cancer Center;

---

12 American Cancer Society Cancer Action Network, *Barriers to Patient Enrollment in Therapeutic Clinical Trials for Cancer: A Landscape Report,* 2018. Accessed June 7, 2021 https://www.fightcancer.org/policy-resources/barriers-patient-enrollment-therapeutic-clinic al-trials-cancer.

13 Food and Drug Administration, *2015-2019 Drug Trials Snapshot: Summary Report,* November 2020.

and VA. The agencies may award funds to researchers outside of the federal government through a competitive process whereby researchers submit grant applications to the funding agency, or they may provide those funds to agency researchers within the federal government to conduct the trials. For some agencies, competitive grants may be renewed by the agencies, sometimes requiring a renewal application. CDMRP, on the other hand, requires that all research funding be openly competed, so those wishing to apply for follow-on or additional funding must submit new applications to be evaluated through a review process.

NIH

NIH's NCI is the federal government's principal agency for cancer research and training. NCI has 30 divisions, offices, and centers that work together on its cancer research agenda and the institute supports trials through a number of different trial networks and programs. For example, NCI supports the National Clinical Trials Network, a collection of organizations and clinicians that coordinates and supports cancer clinical trials at more than 2,200 sites worldwide. NCI also supports the NCI Community Oncology Research Program, a national network of sites that expands the reach of the National Clinical Trials Network and provides infrastructure for conducting clinical trials focused on cancer prevention, screening, supportive care and symptom management, surveillance, health-related quality of life, and cancer care delivery. These sites then operate more than 1,000 research sites to bring cancer clinical trials and care delivery studies to people in their own communities. In fiscal year 2021, NCI received $6.35 billion in funding.

DOD

DOD has two primary organizations that fund cancer research.

- CDMRP originated via a Congressional appropriation in 1992 to foster novel approaches to biomedical research. CDMRP is located within the U.S. Army Medical Research and Development Command, which is the largest medical research enterprise within DOD. CDMRP administers research programs targeting specific cancers or cancer topics as directed by

Congress. Awards of these CDMRP funds must be openly competed and may be made to both DOD and non-DOD organizations. In fiscal year 2022, CDMRP received $1.54 billion in appropriations for all 35 of its research program areas. Of those funds, $585 million were directed to its 10 cancer research program areas; however, these funds support more than just clinical trials.

- John P. Murtha Cancer Center at the Walter Reed National Military Medical Center is the DOD Cancer Center of Excellence. DOD provides $30 million in direct funding to Murtha Cancer Center to conduct state-of-the-art clinical care and innovative research, including clinical trials for the military and its beneficiaries.

VA

VA's Office of Research and Development has a strategic priority to increase veterans' access to high-quality clinical trials. Within VA's Office of Research and Development, the VA Cooperative Studies Program plans and conducts large, multicenter clinical trials and epidemiological studies, including those for cancer. The Cooperative Studies Program received more than $104 million in funding in fiscal year 2021.

Federal Agencies with Roles Other Than Funding or Conducting Clinical Trials

FDA, NIH, and CMS, all within HHS, have a role related to clinical trials other than funding or conducting trials. This includes the issuance of guidance and regulations, and development of policies for those conducting clinical trials.

- One of FDA's roles is to help ensure the safety and efficacy of drugs. It does so by reviewing applications for new drugs, and issuing guidance and regulations related to the study of drugs, including clinical trials.

- NIH issues guidance and policies related to the conduct of clinical trials it funds. (A list of FDA and NIH guidance and policy related to diversity in clinical trials is in app. II.)
- Since 2000, CMS has paid for routine patient care costs for Medicare beneficiaries participating in clinical trials.[14] Generally, CMS defines routine costs as those items or services provided to an individual under a qualifying clinical trial, including those provided to diagnose or treat complications resulting from participation in the trial, if they would have been otherwise covered outside of the trial.
- CMS also pays for routine patient care costs for Medicaid beneficiaries participating in clinical trials.[15] In December 2020, a law was enacted requiring Medicaid coverage of routine costs associated with clinical trial participation.[16] Prior to this, states had flexibility to limit such coverage, and some states chose not to cover such services. As of January 2022, states are required to cover routine costs associated with participation in clinical trials.

Barriers Affecting Patient Enrollment in Cancer Trials

The multitude of barriers that affect the enrollment of patients into clinical trials has been described in published research. Some of the barriers frequently mentioned include the following.

- Unconscious bias. Unconscious bias is when stereotypes or cultural concepts influence behavior without realization. Unconscious bias can influence all stages of the clinical trial process, beginning with which patients are told about the availability of a clinical trial. One report found that this bias, based on misconceptions or assumptions about race, ethnicity, socioeconomic status, or other patient

---

[14] Medicare is the federally financed health insurance program for persons aged 65 and over, certain individuals with disabilities, and individuals with end-stage renal disease.

[15] Medicaid is a joint federal-state health care financing program for certain low-income and medically needed individuals.

[16] Consolidated Appropriations Act, 2021, Pub. L. No, 116-260, div. CC, tit. II, § 210, 134 Stat. 1182, 2989-92.

characteristics can affect a health care provider's decision to mention the option of clinical trial participation to a patient.[17]

- Mistrust and historical discrimination. Research has shown that many patients from underrepresented racial and ethnic groups have a general mistrust of medical research stemming from historical and contemporary instances of racism and research misconduct.[18] Research has shown that a lack trust in research, investigators, and the research system, and fear of being treated "as a guinea pig" can be a barrier to participation in clinical trials.[19]
- Location. A clinical trial's location may also be a barrier for a variety of reasons. First, clinical trials are often at major cancer centers or other sites where individuals from traditionally underrepresented groups are less likely to receive care, and may not be near where certain patients live.[20] For example, one study assessing the economic burden of cancer patients in early-phase clinical trials from a cancer center in Houston, Texas, found that half of the patients studied lived more than 300 miles from the clinic conducting the trial, and another 27 percent lived more than 101 miles away.[21]

---

[17] Case Comprehensive Cancer Center, "*Unconscious Bias: An Introduction*" (Cleveland, OH: Case Western University, 2015), accessed December 16, 2021, https://case.edu/cancer/research/clinical-research-office/minority-accrual-committee/cultural-inclusion and-awareness/unconscious-bias-introduction.

[18] M. Awidi and S. A. Hadidi, "Participation of Black Americans in Cancer Clinical Trials: Current Challenges and Proposed Solutions," *JCO Oncology Practice,* vol. 17, no. 5 (2021); B. Nazha, M. Mishra, R. Pentz, and T. K. Owonikoko, "Enrollment of Racial Minorities in Clinical Trials: Old Problem Assumes New Urgency in the Age of Immunotherapy," *ASCO Educational Book* (2019). J. G. Ford et al., "Barriers to Recruiting Underrepresented Populations to Cancer Clinical Trials: A Systematic Review," *Cancer,* vol. 112, no. 2 (2008).

[19] B. E. Bierer et al., *Achieving Diversity.*

[20] See Awidi and Hadidi, "Participation of Black Americans;" American Society of Clinical Oncology, *Improving Diversity in Clinical Trial Participation: Policy Brief,* (Oct. 2020), accessed July 7, 2022, https://www.asco.org/sites/new-www.asco.org/files/content-files/advocacy-and-policy/docu ments/2020-CTDiv-Brief.pdf; J. M. Unger et al., "Systematic Review and Meta-Analysis of the Magnitude of Structural, Clinical, and Physician and Patient Barriers to Cancer Clinical Trial Participation." *JNCI: Journal of the National Cancer Institute* Vol. 111 (2019), 245- 255.

[21] Early-phase clinical trials are the first tests of a particular treatment and usually involve small groups of people. R. W. Huey et al.,"Patient-Reported Out-of-Pocket Costs and Financial Toxicity During Early-Phase Oncology Clinical Trials," *The Oncologist,* vol. 26 (2021).

For many reasons, it may be important to have trials be conducted where patients and caregivers are in order to improve awareness, access, and trust, all of which have been cited as barriers to participation.[22]

Availability of prostate cancer trials by county and population

One study of Black men—whose incidence rate of prostate cancer is 70 percent greater than that of White men and whose mortality rate is 2.5 times higher than White men— looked at availability of prostate cancer clinical trials by county and population. It found that the counties with a higher proportion of Blacks were less likely to have access to both cancer facilities and prostate cancer trials.

Source: W-J. Wang, S. D. Ramsey, C. S. Bennette, and A. Bansal, "Racial Disparities in Access to Prostate Cancer Clinical Trials" A County-Level Analysis." *JNCI Cancer Spectrum*, vol. 6, no. 1 (2022). | GAO-23-105245.

Importance of location and setting

One study reported engaging Black patients in health interventions in community barbershops or predominately Black-serving churches was a key to success. The authors noted that the locations provided the patients with a familiar setting and trusted individuals and that location convenience was essential.

Source: C. R. Rogers et al., "Barriers to and Facilitators of Recruitment of Adult African American Men for Colorectal Cancer Research: An Instrumental Exploratory Case Study," *JCO Oncology Practice*, vo. 17, no. 5 (2021) | GAO-23-105245.

- Inclusion and exclusion criteria. A clinical trial's inclusion and exclusion criteria —the factors that determine whether a patient is eligible to participate—may have bias embedded in them. Such criteria might include biological factors that result in bias toward certain individuals. For example, some of these eligibility factors (such as blood pressure) may vary between racial and ethnic groups and may therefore result in the exclusion of certain groups.
- *Cultural competence, linguistic, and literacy factors.* Cultural competence includes understanding and respect of the diversity of a patient population, including factors such as language,

[22] The Deloitte Center for Health Solutions and Pharmaceutical Research and Manufacturers of America, "Enhancing Clinical Trial Diversity: Stakeholder Perspectives on Advancing Research Through Representative Clinical Trials" (2021).

communication styles, beliefs, attitudes and behaviors. Having staff of a trial that shares cultural characteristics with the patients can facilitate participation.[23] Other barriers have to do with language. For example, the language used in consent forms can be difficult for patients to understand. Further, trial materials may not be offered in the native language of a patient. At the same time, some have noted that translating consent forms can be costly and those costs are rarely covered in research budgets.[24]

- *Costs and other logistical barriers.* The costs of participating in a clinical trial can reduce a patient's ability to enroll or continue participating. Such costs include:
  - Investigational care costs are costs associated with the drug being studied and related services that would not otherwise be required such as blood tests for safety data and are covered by the sponsor of the clinical trial.
  - Routine care costs are direct medical costs for those services that would have been provided to a patient even without their participation in a clinical trial such as services for therapy or prevention of complications. These costs are typically covered by insurance, or if denied by insurance or the patient lacks insurance, by the patient themselves.
  - The third type of costs are nonmedical, out-of-pocket costs, such as lodging and meals, transportation, and dependent care or childcare. These costs are typically the responsibility of the patient.

Lessons in cultural competence

One study identified lessons learned with increasing participation of American Indian/Alaska Natives in genetic research that can increase diverse representation in another research. Understanding that a lack of cultural competence can be a barrier, the authors recommended approaches that use cultural sensitivity to foster trust through the following:

- Becoming familiar with tribal governance and structure because each tribe is unique and culturally distinct

---

[23] Bierer et al., Achieving Diversity.

[24] J. M. Kahn et al., "Strategies to Improve Diversity, Equity, and Inclusion in Clinical Trials," Cancer, (Jan. 15, 2022).

- Building trust with the community by learning the tribe's history of involvement with research; including by spending time in the community, and engaging stakeholders throughout the research process
- Becoming culturally attuned
- Being straightforward with expectations and ideal communication strategies
- Developing a research agreement and plan for using data
- Ensuring the study is review by the tribe for ethical and cultural considerations
- Providing the tribe with resources and personnel to support the study
- Balancing the need for scientific knowledge with the benefit to the community

Source: D. M. Carroll et al., "Recommendations to Researchers for Aiding in Increasing American Indian Representation in Genetic Research and Personalized Medicine," Personalized Medicine, vol. 18, no. 1 (2021). | GAO-23-105245.

Logistical barriers that have indirect costs for patients include the time commitment, loss of income, and family considerations. As certain racial and ethnic groups are affected more by lower incomes and are more likely to have jobs based on an hourly wage, these costs make it harder for them to fit clinical trial participation into their schedule. However, many trials do not provide reimbursement for nonmedical costs of participating in a trial because of concerns that reimbursement for costs may be seen as an inducement to participation in a clinical trial.

Out-of-pocket costs

One study found that overall, 48 percent of the patients in cancer clinical trials had monthly out-of-pocket costs of at least $1,000. They also found that patients used a variety source to pay those costs including using savings, withdrawing money from retirement accounts, borrowing money from friends and family, having a fundraiser, and working extra hours or an additional job.

Source: R. W. Huey et al., "Patient-Reported Out-of-Pocket Costs and Financial Toxicity During Early-Phase Oncology Clinical Trials," *The Oncologist*, vol. 26 (2021). | GAO-23- 105245.

A Range of Federal Actions Focus on Enrolling a Diverse Group of Patients in Cancer Clinical Trials

DOD, HHS, and VA are engaged in a range of actions that facilitate enrollment of a diverse group of patients in federally funded cancer clinical trials. These actions include developing research collaborations, modifying research practices, reducing barriers to patient participation, and collecting and sharing data. (See fig. 1 for a summary of federal actions within each category.)

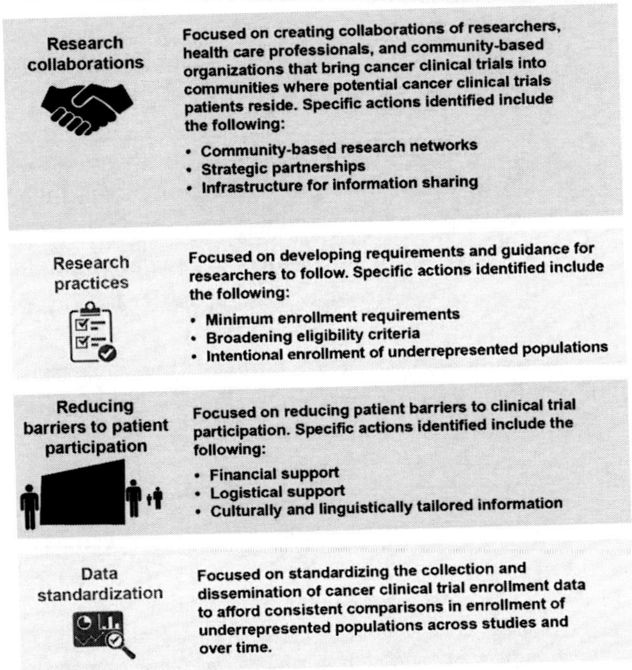

Source: GAO analysis of information from the Department of Defense, Department of Health and Human Services, and Department of Veterans Affairs. | GAO-23-105245.

Figure 1. Categories of Federal Actions to Facilitate Enrollment of a Diverse Group of Patients in Cancer Clinical Trials.

Federal Actions Focused on Research Collaborations

According to agency officials and reviews of agency documentation, federal agencies have created collaborations of researchers, health care professionals, and community-based organizations that bring cancer clinical trials into communities where potential patients from underrepresented populations live. These collaborations have (1) created research networks in the communities where patients live, (2) developed strategic partnerships with institutions serving patients from underrepresented populations, and (3) established an infrastructure for researchers to collaborate and share information.

Community-based research networks. NCI and VA have created networks of multiple clinical trial research sites placed within communities, which can enable sustained community interaction that has been shown to build trust and establish meaningful relationships with patients. Interacting directly with communities fosters the input of community stakeholders, which can help clinical trial teams incorporate community feedback into research design and identify individuals and organizations that can help facilitate the enrollment of a diverse group of patients in cancer clinical trials. Examples of community-based networks include the following:

- The NCI Community Oncology Research Program is a national network of seven research bases that provide scientific and statistical leadership in developing, implementing, and analyzing clinical trials. The program also includes 46 community sites that bring cancer clinical trials to patients in their own communities. One of the goals of the program is to bring clinical research studies to patients in their own communities so the evidence generated from clinical trials can contribute to improved patient outcomes for all people. One feature of the program is that 14 of the 46 sites are Minority/Underserved Community Sites, which are those for which at least 30 percent of the patient population is comprised of racial and ethnic groups other than non-Hispanic White or rural residents. The program enrolls patients in NCI-supported clinical trials at approximately 1,000 affiliate hospitals and cancer centers.
- The NCI and VA Interagency Group to Accelerate Trials Enrollment partnership between NCI and VA facilitates enrollment of veterans with cancer, including patients from diverse backgrounds, into NCI-funded clinical trials. This partnership helps bring NCI clinical trials to VA patients so that they do not have to seek treatment outside of the VA health care system. The goal is to build the capacity of VA Medical Centers with dedicated staffing and sustainable infrastructure so they can offer NCI clinical trials in the future. VA officials stated that this structure provides local support, which can

help VA Medical Centers identify site-specific challenges related to clinical trial execution.

Strategic partnerships. DOD, FDA, and NCI have established strategic partnerships with organizations serving underrepresented populations, including health care and educational institutions and consumer advocacy organizations. Research has shown that the goal of these partnerships is to create collaborations with organizations already working with patient communities to build trust and design clinical trials that are more inclusive of underrepresented communities. Examples of federal strategic partnerships include the following:

- According to officials, cancer programs managed by DOD's CDMRP have encouraged multi-institutional collaboration with institutions and outreach programs at university hospitals, cancer treatment centers, and minority-serving institutions. These types of collaborations may help increase diversity in the research community, which can reduce barriers affecting enrollment of certain underrepresented populations. Some CDMRP-funded cancer researchers also partner with patient advocates and consumer advocacy organizations throughout the clinical trial enrollment process to develop relationships and build trust. Some CDMRP cancer funding opportunities require such partnerships.
- FDA's Oncology Center of Excellence conducts an initiative called Project Equity to promote research practices and policies that facilitate enrollment of a diverse group of patients.[25] It does this through outreach and partnerships with oncology stakeholders, including academic organizations, pharmaceutical sponsors, regulatory agencies, and professional organizations. FDA officials stated that collaborations with stakeholders through Project Equity have explored ways to improve trial design and trial conduct that can generate clinical trial results across a diverse group of patients.
- NCI's Center to Reduce Cancer Health Disparities oversees the Partnerships to Advance Cancer Health Equity program that provides institutional awards for the development of partnerships between NCI- designated cancer centers and institutions focused on

---

25 See https://www.fda.gov/about-fda/oncology-center-excellence/project-equity, accessed August 10, 2022.

underrepresented populations. NCI officials stated that the partnerships are focused on increasing cancer research education for students and improving the effectiveness of cancer care in underserved communities. The program establishes partnerships through two funding mechanisms, one directly supporting researchers and one focused on building long-term relationships with institutions.

Infrastructure for information sharing. DOD, NCI, and VA research networks provide an infrastructure for network members to share information, such as best practices for enrolling patients from underrepresented populations and feedback to clinical trial administrators. Examples of federal actions in this area include the following:

- Murtha Cancer Center officials told us that the center has an Oversight Committee comprised of senior leadership and external federal experts from VA and NCI that reviews clinical trial participation data and provides trial recommendations based on their findings. The Oversight Committee has made recommendations for ensuring the proper inclusion of eligible military and veteran patients. Agencies officials noted they serve populations with high proportions of persons from racial and ethnic groups other than non-Hispanic White.
- NIH officials stated that the NCI Community Oncology Research Program's seven research bases and the NCI National Clinical Trials Network membership organizations each hold periodic meetings, which serve as a forum for NCI officials and local researchers to share research best practices that address clinical trial participation gaps.[26]
- VA officials stated that the NCI and VA Interagency Group to Accelerate Trials Enrollment program coordinates clinical trial researchers by hosting monthly conference calls, sharing information via newsletters, and providing central logistical support. This allows researchers to share issues with trial administrators as they arise. For example, researchers and officials learned through these information-sharing meetings that existing trial inclusion and exclusion criteria often restricts participation of those with hearing loss, more common

[26] The National Clinical Trials Network consists of four adult cancer groups, one group focused solely on childhood cancers, and a Canadian Collaborating Clinical Trials Network.

in veterans. VA officials were able to escalate this issue to NCI in an effort to make trial eligibility criteria more inclusive.

Federal Actions Focused on Research Practices

Federal agencies have undertaken actions to modify research practices with the goal of increasing the enrollment of a diverse group of patients. Federal actions include making recommendations for clinical trials researchers on setting minimum requirements for clinical trial enrollment, broadening patient eligibility criteria, and intentional enrollment of underrepresented populations.

Minimum enrollment requirements. The DOD CDMRP's prostate and kidney cancer programs require consortium-led clinical trials to enroll a minimum of 5 percent of their patients from a diverse background, which includes factors such as race, geography, and socioeconomic status.

DOD officials stated the programs monitor planned and actual enrollment annually through technical progress reports submitted by researchers.

CDMRP officials noted that while there is no penalty for network sites that do not meet the 5 percent minimum, the minimum percentage provides encouragement to researchers to focus on enrollment of patients from diverse backgrounds. CDMRP officials told us that nine of 10 sites in the consortium have exceeded the 5 percent minimum enrollment of patients from underrepresented populations, with enrollment ranging from 9 to 42 percent.[27] For network sites under the minimum, CDMRP science officers meet with researchers and discuss strategies to increase enrollment for underrepresented groups.

Broadening eligibility criteria. FDA and NCI have developed guidance for researchers for developing inclusion and exclusion criteria that facilitate enrollment of a diverse group of patients. Broadening eligibility criteria can increase the potential pool of clinical trial patients, particularly those from diverse backgrounds, such as older adults and those from certain racial and ethnic groups historically underrepresented in clinical trials, without affecting the safety of patients or effectiveness of the trial.

FDA published guidance in 2020 to help facilitate the broadening of eligibility criteria so that patients enrolled in trials will better reflect the

[27] The only Clinical Consortium site under 5 percent had an underrepresented enrollment rate of 3.7 percent.

population most likely to use the drug if it is approved.[28] The guidance recommended research practices that include to avoid unnecessarily excluding patients, to adapt research studies based on ongoing findings, and to recruit patients with different levels of disease severity. As a result, this guidance promotes understanding of important safety and effectiveness information for all patients who may benefit from the drug after approval. FDA also published guidance regarding the inclusion of older adults in cancer clinical trials.[29]

NCI, using recommendations from the American Society of Clinical Oncology and Friends of Cancer Research, developed guidance, effective as of 2018, that includes recommendations for researchers to broaden clinical trial eligibility related to patients with multiple medical conditions and adolescent patients.[30] NCI merged these recommendations into a Generic Protocol Template that some NCI funding programs require clinical trials to use when developing eligibility criteria. NCI added additional criteria to the guidelines in response to recommendations made in May 2021 by American Society of Clinical Oncology and Friends of Cancer Research that sought to identify additional criteria that can pose significant barriers to clinical trial enrollment.[31]

Intentional enrollment of underrepresented populations. DOD, FDA, NIH, and VA have implemented practices that support strategies for enrolling a more diverse group of patients in clinical trials. Research has shown that considering recruitment goals and strategies for enrolling underrepresented populations early in a clinical trial can improve the effectiveness of increasing

---

[28] Food and Drug Administration, Center for Drug Evaluation and Research and Center for Biologics Evaluation and Research, Enhancing the Diversity of Clinical Trial Populations — Eligibility Criteria, Enrollment Practices, and Trial Designs, Guidance for Industry (Silver Spring, Md.: Nov. 2020).

[29] Food and Drug Administration, Inclusion of Older Adults in Cancer Clinical Trials – Guidance for Industry. (Silver Spring, Md.: Mar. 2022).

[30] National Cancer Institute, Cancer Therapy Evaluation Program, *Broadening/Modernizing Eligibility Criteria for National Cancer Institute (NCI) Sponsored Clinical Trials* (Bethesda, Md.: Dec. 2021). The continued use of commonly accepted eligibility criteria has been found to exclude certain populations (e.g., racial and ethnic groups other than non-Hispanic White, older adults) without strong clinical or scientific justification.

[31] The American Society for Clinical Oncology and Friends of Cancer Research published a paper that recommends the broadening of additional eligibility criteria. The recommendations seek to promote the inclusion of all populations who are anticipated to benefit from a therapy while excluding patients only where safety concerns warrant exclusion of patients with certain characteristics. See E. S. Kim et al., "Continuing to Broaden Eligibility Criteria to Make Clinical Trials More Representative and Inclusive: ASCO–Friends of Cancer Research Joint Research Statement," *Clinical Cancer Research*, vol. 27, no. 9 (2021): 2394-2399.

the enrollment of those patients.[32] Some agencies have required researchers to include intentional enrollment strategies as a separate attachment to their funding applications. In addition, VA has provided a toolkit to help research teams incorporate these strategies into their clinical trials.

Since October 2020, DOD's CDMRP policy has required all applicants for clinical research funding to submit a proposed strategy for the recruitment of women and underrepresented populations, including enrollment estimates by sex and race/ethnicity, at the time they apply. CDMRP officials told us they created the requirement as a separate attachment in most of the funding opportunities to stress the importance of this part of the application.

- Murtha Cancer Center officials stated that the center's strategy to promote diversity and equity in DOD cancer studies directs research consent staff who are hired to enroll patients into clinical trials to prioritize recruitment of underrepresented groups. Finally, the strategy tasks administrative research staff to review incoming cancer patients from racial and ethnic groups other than non-Hispanic White, identify those who would be eligible for clinical trials, and purposefully approach these patients to determine their interest in participating.
- FDA developed draft guidance in April 2022 with recommendations that clinical trial researchers and funders develop race and ethnicity diversity plans.[33] The draft guidance recommends that researchers establish enrollment goals based on the population of patients who will use the treatment, details strategies to enroll and retain patients from diverse backgrounds, and describes how differences in safety and effectiveness can be assessed by race and ethnicity.
- NIH's two inclusion policies require funding applicants to submit inclusion enrollment plans as a component of the application.[34] The

---

[32] S. H. Javid et al., "A prospective analysis of the influence of older age on physician and patient decision-making when considering enrollment in breast cancer clinical trials," *Oncologist*, vol. 17, no. 9 (2012):1180–1190.

[33] Food and Drug Administration, Diversity Plans to Improve Enrollment of Participants from Underrepresented Racial and Ethnic Populations in Clinical Trials Guidance for Industry, Draft Guidance (Silver Spring, Md.: Apr. 2022); the 60-day comment period ended on June 13, 2022, and FDA officials said that when final, this guidance will reflect FDA's current thinking on this topic.

[34] National Institutes of Health, NIH Policy and Guidelines on the Inclusion of Women and Minorities as Subjects in Clinical Research (Bethesda, Md.: Oct. 2001); National Institutes of Health, Revision: NIH Policy and Guidelines on the Inclusion of Individuals Across the

first policy states that applications should describe the proposed study population in terms of sex/gender and race/ethnicity. A second similar policy describes recommendations for age. Both policies state that applicants should provide a rationale for the selection. Any exclusion based on sex/gender, race/ethnicity, or age must include a scientific or ethics-based justification.

- VA's Women's Health Research Network, in collaboration with the VA Cooperative Studies Program, developed a toolkit of resources that can be used to better support researchers in enhancing participation of women veterans in clinical trials. The toolkit includes recruitment strategies, approaches to training research staff, and suggestions for local resources to support recruitment of women.

Federal Actions Focused on Reducing Barriers to Patient Participation

CMS, DOD, NCI, VA, and FDA have implemented actions focused on reducing financial, logistical, and cultural and linguistic barriers to patient participation in clinical trials.

Financial support. CMS, DOD, and NCI have taken action to address the financial barriers, which can contribute to low clinical trial participation rates for patients, particularly from underrepresented populations.[35] Agencies' actions to reduce financial barriers for clinical trial patients include compensation for routine costs associated with trial participation and reimbursement of patient out-of-pocket costs, such as transportation and dependent care.

- As previously described, Medicare and Medicaid cover routine patient care costs for beneficiaries participating in qualifying clinical trials. CMS officials stated that since Medicare coverage of such costs began in 2000, local Medicare administrators determine what routine costs are eligible for coverage for each separate qualifying clinical trial. Covered costs are those they deem reasonable and necessary and

---

Lifespan as Participants in Research Involving Human Subjects (Bethesda, Md.: Dec. 2017).

[35] R. D. Nipp et al., "Recognizing the financial burden of cancer patients in clinical trials," *Oncologist*, vol. 20 (2015): 572-575.

that are aligned with costs that would regularly be covered by Medicare.

Federal law required Medicaid coverage of routine patient costs associated with participation in qualifying clinical trials beginning January 1, 2022. According to CMS officials, state Medicaid administrators are responsible for establishing guidelines, within federal parameters, on coverage, reimbursement requirements, and processing reimbursements for costs related to clinical trials. Each state is required to submit a state plan amendment to CMS to implement the new benefit, and, as of June 2022, 44 state plan amendments had been approved.[36] Because Medicaid programs vary by state, Medicaid coverage for services that are within clinical trials also varies by state. CMS officials told us that the biggest challenge that clinical trial researchers may face are these state differences, particularly for those running clinical trials with patients from multiple states. In addition, state Medicaid programs are required to cover non-emergency transportation. According to CMS officials, this benefit covers the costs of necessary transportation for Medicaid-approved care, which includes approved care provided as part of clinical trials, and can cover other related travel expenses, including the cost of meals and lodging.

- According to officials, DOD's CDMRP allows cancer research budgets to cover out-of-pocket patient expenses associated with participation in clinical trials, including transportation, dependent care, food, and lodging. To increase patient awareness of this benefit, CDMRP has encouraged clinical trial researchers to state clearly to patients that these out-of-pocket costs will be reimbursed if they participate in that clinical trial. In addition, DOD's Murtha Cancer Center arranges travel and housing for active duty service members who are undergoing cancer treatment or participating in cancer clinical trials. Officials stated that this benefit allows patients to participate in cancer research without any additional cost to the patient.

---

[36] A Medicaid state plan amendment is an agreement between a state and the federal government describing how that state administers its Medicaid program. The state plan amendment sets out groups of individuals to be covered, services to be provided, methodologies for providers to be reimbursed and the administrative activities that are underway in the state. When a state is planning to make a change to its program policies or operational approach, states send state plan amendments to CMS for review and approval.

- According to officials, NCI's Center for Cancer Research provides support to trial participants for travel expenses, food, lodging, and inpatient and outpatient medical treatment.[37] For example, NCI provides free lodging on the NIH campus for certain qualifying patients.

Logistical support. FDA, NCI, and VA have taken action to address logistical barriers, such as time commitments and distant research locations, which have been shown to deter patients from participating in clinical trials.[38] Related agency actions, which began in response to the COVID-19 pandemic, include using telemedicine for routine visits, shipping study medications to patients, and using local clinics and imaging centers for certain activities.

- FDA issued guidance that highlighted existing flexibilities for alternative locations or research processes for clinical trial activities, such as local imaging centers, virtual visits, and delivery of study medications that researchers could take during the COVID-19 pandemic.[39] This guidance is designed to help industry, researchers, and institutional review boards protect patient safety and facilitate continuing research. The guidance is in effect for the duration of the COVID-19 public health emergency, though agency officials said they could extend it beyond that date if needed. In 2022, FDA published draft guidance on using digital health technology to obtain data remotely from participants in clinical trials.[40]
- NCI issued similar interim guidance that created flexibilities for continued clinical trial research during the COVID-19 pandemic.[41] The interim guidance included alternative procedures, such as

[37] The Center for Cancer Research is the largest division of NCI's intramural research program with nearly 250 basic and clinical research groups located on the NIH campus.

[38] E. D., Giarelli et al., "Research participation among Asian American women at risk for cervical cancer: Exploratory pilot of barriers and enhancers," *Journal of Immigrant and Minority Health*, vol. 13, no. 6 (2011):1055–1068.

[39] Food and Drug Administration, Conduct of Clinical Trials of Medical Products during the COVID-19 Public Health Emergency — Guidance for Industry, Investigators, and Institutional Review Boards (Silver Spring, Md.: Aug. 2021).

[40] Food and Drug Administration, Digital Health Technologies for Remote Data Acquisition in Clinical Investigation (Draft Guidance for Industry, investigators, and Other Stakeholders), (Silver Spring, Md.: Jan. 2022).

[41] National Cancer Institute, Interim Guidance for Patients on Clinical Trials Supported by the NCI Cancer Therapy Evaluation Program and the NCI Community Oncology Research Program (NCORP) (Bethesda, Md., Mar. 2020).

allowing shipment of study medications to patients and clarifying how researchers could work with local health care providers to perform certain trial activities. NCI officials stated that the agency is working to create permanent recommendations for these new processes.

- VA officials stated that researchers have incorporated telehealth in clinical trials to engage more veterans living in rural areas and reduce the burden of physically visiting a VA medical center. VA expanded telehealth into clinical trials as a way to enable continued patients' participation during the COVID-19 pandemic. VA has also made efforts to ship study medications to patients' homes to reduce the burden of traveling to a medical center. Stakeholders from a cancer advocacy association and a pharmaceutical company told us that continuing the use of telehealth may allow patients to overcome logistical barriers making it less burdensome to participate.

Culturally and linguistically tailored information. FDA and NIH have implemented actions to support developing culturally and linguistically appropriate materials to facilitate enrollment of a diverse group of patients in clinical trials. Research has shown that educational materials in different languages, with culturally relevant messages and images and clear language, are important in increasing the enrollment of patients across many racial and ethnic backgrounds.[42] Examples of federal actions to address cultural and linguistic barriers include the following:

- FDA issued guidance on enhancing clinical trial diversity that includes recommendations for practices that increase cultural inclusiveness.[43] Recommendations include providing researcher cultural competency training and providing trial resources and documents in multiple languages and multilingual research staff and/or interpreters in order to encourage the participation and retention of individuals with limited English comprehension.
- NCI's National Outreach Network employs community health educators at 24 NCI-designated cancer centers to develop and disseminate culturally appropriate, evidence-based, cancer information tailored to the specific needs and expectations of

---

[42] National Academies of Sciences, Engineering, and Medicine. Improving Representation.
[43] Food and Drug Administration, *Enhancing the Diversity of Clinical Trial Populations.*

underrepresented populations. For example, the Beckman Research Institute's City of Hope National Outreach Network program seeks to increase community knowledge of importance of clinical trials in ethnic minority communities, specifically Latino, African American, and Chinese. (See fig. 2.)

- According to officials, NIH developed "plain English" consent forms for clinical trial participation to reduce potential language barriers.[44]

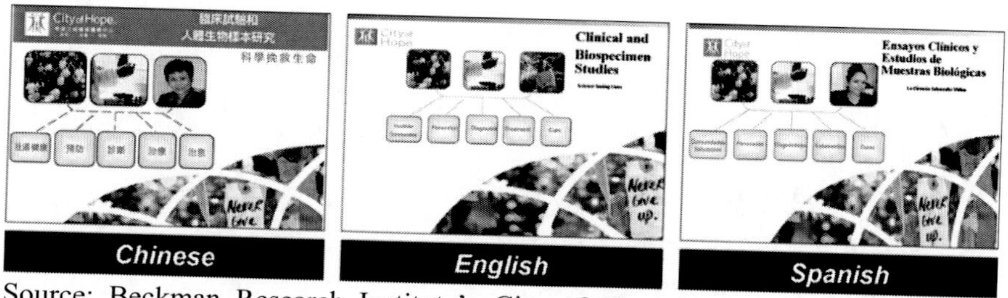

Source: Beckman Research Institute's City of Hope National Outreach Network Program. | GAO-23-105245.

Figure 2. Clinical Trial Educational Materials Translated and Culturally Adapted through NCI's National Outreach Network.

Federal Actions Focused on Data Standardization

DOD, FDA, NIH, and VA have implemented processes to standardize the collection of demographic data about clinical trial patients, which allows agencies to analyze results more effectively for patients from diverse backgrounds. Examples of federal actions include the following:

- DOD's CDMRP implemented a policy in October 2020 requiring clinical trial researchers to use a standardized form to submit data annually about the demographics of the patients they enrolled in clinical trials. According to DOD officials, this form allows researchers to report information on patient demographics, including sex, race, and ethnicity to track progress in meeting the clinical study's patient recruitment goals.

[44] This effort aligns with work by the Plain Language Action and Information Network—a working group of federal employees from different agencies and specialties—that developed the Federal Plain Language Guidelines to assist agencies in developing documents with clear communication.

- FDA released guidance in 2016 to standardize the collection of demographic data in clinical trials.[45] The guidance established a standardized framework for consistency in the definition of race and ethnicity data.
- As stated in NIH policy, each NIH institute or center, including NCI, collects and reviews sex and gender, race, and ethnicity enrollment data, which are compiled as part of annual reports.[46] According to officials, NCI creates a triennial report using these data that describes enrollment in supported clinical research by sex and race/ethnicity.
- According to officials, all studies funded by VA's Cooperative Studies Program—VA's primary multisite clinical trial funding program—use a standard data collection template, which includes age, sex, location, and race/ethnicity.
- According to officials, all studies funded by VA's Cooperative Studies Program—VA's primary multisite clinical trial funding program—use a standard data collection template, which includes age, sex, location, and race/ethnicity.

Selected Cancer Centers Used a Variety of Practices to Facilitate Enrollment of Patients from Diverse Backgrounds in Cancer Clinical Trials

The 17 non-federal cancer centers in our review have implemented a variety of practices designed to facilitate enrollment of patients from diverse backgrounds in cancer clinical trials. These practices fall into four categories: (1) organization-level practices, (2) community-level practices, (3) workforce-level practices, and (4) patient-level practices. Figure 2 describes the practices in each category.[47] Of the 17 cancer centers we reviewed, 15 centers noted

---

[45] Food and Drug Administration, Guidance on Collection of Race and Ethnicity Data in Clinical Trials (Silver Spring, Md.: Oct. 2016).

[46] National Institutes of Health, NIH Policy and Guidelines on the Inclusion of Women and Minorities.

[47] These four categories generally align with categories identified in published literature. See, for example: O. Garrick, et al., "Advancing Inclusive Research: Establishing Collaborative Strategies to Improve Diversity in Clinical Trials." *Ethnicity & Disease*, vol. 32, no. 1 (2022); J. M. Regnante et al., "US Cancer Centers of Excellence Strategies for Increased Inclusion of Racial and Ethnic Minorities in Clinical Trials." *Journal of Oncology Practice,* vol. 15, no. 4 (2019); American Cancer Society Cancer Action Network, *Barriers to Patient Enrollment in Therapeutic Clinical Trials for Cancer: A Landscape Report,* (2018); and A.

implementing practices in at least three of the four categories.[48] (A description of selected cancer centers can be found in appendix III.)[49]

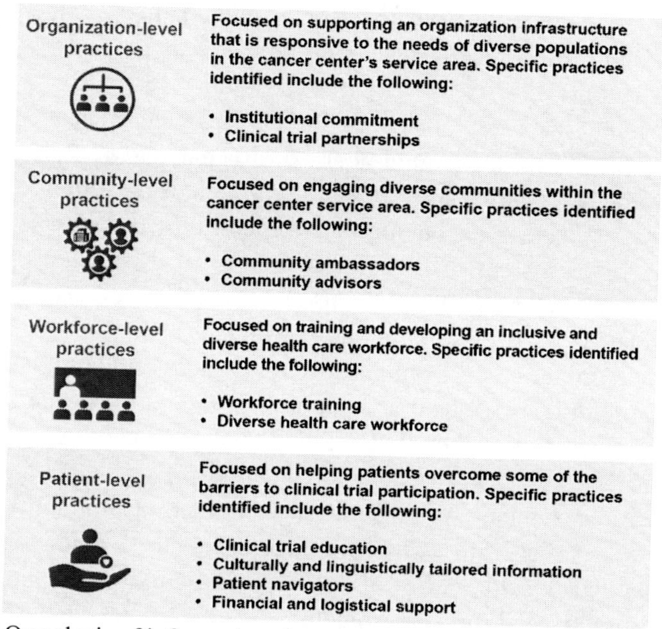
Organization-level practices
Focused on supporting an organization infrastructure that is responsive to the needs of diverse populations in the cancer center's service area. Specific practices identified include the following:
• Institutional commitment
• Clinical trial partnerships
Community-level practices
Focused on engaging diverse communities within the cancer center service area. Specific practices identified include the following:
• Community ambassadors
• Community advisors
Workforce-level practices
Focused on training and developing an inclusive and diverse health care workforce. Specific practices identified include the following:
• Workforce training
• Diverse health care workforce
Patient-level practices
Focused on helping patients overcome some of the barriers to clinical trial participation. Specific practices identified include the following:
• Clinical trial education
• Culturally and linguistically tailored information
• Patient navigators
• Financial and logistical support

Source: GAO analysis of information about the 17 selected cancer centers. | GAO-23-105245.

Figure 3. Categories of Practices to Facilitate Diverse Patient Representation in Cancer Clinical Trials at Selected Cancer Centers.

Organization-Level Practices

We found that all 17 selected cancer centers we reviewed noted implementing organization-level practices to help them understand the needs of diverse

M. Denicoff et al., "The National Cancer Institute-American Society of Clinical Oncology Cancer Trial Accrual Symposium: Summary and Recommendations." *Journal of Oncology Practice*, vol. 9, no. 6 (2013).

48 Our review of the 17 selected cancer centers is based on our analysis of the descriptions provided by the 13 cancer centers that responded to a questionnaire we sent and publicly available information. For our review of the four cancer centers that did not respond to our questionnaire, we relied on publicly available information such as published literature and information available on the centers' websites.

49 Appendix III includes descriptions of the 13 cancer centers that responded to a questionnaire we sent to the 17 cancer centers we identified.

populations within their service area and enhance their ability to enroll a diverse patient population into cancer clinical trials.[50] Specifically, selected cancer centers have noted adoption of an institutional commitment to serving diverse populations in their service area or establishment of partnerships with other organizations to conduct or support clinical trials to increase access for diverse populations.

Institutional commitment. Fourteen of the 17 selected cancer centers noted adopting an institutional commitment to diversity and serving diverse communities in their service area, including through cancer clinical trials. We found that centers have noted having a stated commitment to diversity in their mission and vision statements or strategic plans, or establishing leadership roles and programs, or initiatives focused on helping centers identify and address the needs of diverse communities in their service area. Research suggests that commitments from institutional leaders and infrastructure to support community engagement are important to identifying and addressing the research needs of communities and the barriers relevant to underserved communities.[51]

One example of this is Abramson Cancer Center's Community Outreach and Engagement Program, which is dedicated to helping the Center understand and address the needs of communities in the service area and has developed programs and strategies to help overcome barriers to the enrollment of patients with diverse backgrounds in cancer clinical trials. In 2014, the Center, through the Community Outreach and Engagement Program, implemented a 5-year initiative to increase the enrollment of Black patients into cancer clinical trials. As part of the initiative, the Center promoted clinical trials that address the cancer burden experienced by Black residents within the service area, required that each trial have a plan to recruit Black patients, developed marketing materials tailored to Black patients, and established a partnership with a transportation company to address transportation barriers. The efforts reached more than 10,000 individuals in communities across the service area and, by 2018, had more than doubled the Center's enrollment of Black patients in cancer clinical trials, according to Center officials.

Clinical trial partnerships. Eleven of the 17 selected cancer centers noted establishing partnerships with other organizations to conduct or support clinical trials. Clinical trial partnerships are intended to help centers develop

[50] The term "service area" refers to the geographical *area* served by a cancer center.

[51] National Academies of Sciences, Engineering, and Medicine, *Improving Representation in Clinical Trials and Research Groups*.

and implement strategies to increase diverse participation in clinical trials, or make clinical trials more accessible to patients from diverse backgrounds by, for instance, expanding the number and types of locations that conduct trials. Examples of clinical trial partnerships at the selected cancer centers include the following:

- The Benefis Sletten Cancer Institute is a member of the Montana Cancer Consortium, a clinical trial partnership that receives funding through the NCI Community Oncology Research Program. According to Institute officials, participating in the Montana Cancer Consortium enables the Institute to offer NCI trials to patients in its service area, which includes patients from rural and American Indian communities. Within the Institutes' service area, there are three reservations and one federally recognized landless tribe. Collectively, members of the Montana Cancer Consortium serve underrepresented communities across Montana, Idaho, and Wyoming—communities that previously had little access to clinical trials due to the vastness of the geography and a lack of academic treatment and research facilities. Since it was established in 1995, the Montana Cancer Consortium has enrolled more than 4,000 patients to NCI-funded clinical trials.
- In 2008, the University of Illinois at Chicago, Rush University Medical Center, and John H. Stroger Hospital—three neighboring medical centers in Chicago—established a partnership to help ensure that adolescent and young adult patients at all three centers had access to NCI clinical trials and to increase the representation of patients from racial and ethnic minority groups in trials. Under the partnership, the three centers established a unified research team to share resources and manage trial logistics. Prior to 2008, one of the centers did not have access to NCI trials and the number of NCI trials at the other two centers were limited due to a lack of research resources to support their respective programs. Under the partnership, the overall number of cancer patients at the three sites who enrolled in NCI trials increased from 151 during the 6-year period from 2002 through 2008 to 825 during the 9-year period from 2008 through 2017, according to a study analyzing trial enrollment data before and

after the group was formed.[52] The study also found that the percentage of trial patients from a racial and ethnic group other than non-Hispanic White increased from 52 percent to 66 percent during those same time periods. The percentage of adolescent and young adult cancer patients enrolled in trials also increased, from 34 percent to 49 percent during those same time periods.

Community-Level Practices

We found that 13 of the 17 selected cancer centers we reviewed noted implementing practices focused on engaging diverse communities within the cancer center service area. These practices include working with community ambassadors—representatives of the community—to increase awareness of clinical trials and working with community advisors representing diverse community stakeholders to help centers understand and address the needs and perspectives of diverse communities in their service area.

Community ambassadors. Seven of the 17 selected cancer centers noted working with community ambassadors to educate diverse communities on clinical trials and promote clinical trial participation.

Educating communities on the role of clinical trials and the safeguards in place to protect trial participants may help cancer centers overcome some of the barriers to diverse representation in trials, such as a lack of awareness about clinical trials and a fear of participation in trials.

Community ambassadors may serve as trusted messengers for communicating clinical trial information to diverse communities.[53] Examples of community ambassadors at the selected cancer centers include the following:

- The Yale Center for Clinical Investigation, as part of its Cultural Ambassador Program, works with leaders from two community organizations in historically underrepresented communities to help increase enrollment of Hispanic and Black patients in clinical trials.[54]

---

[52] N. Mittal et al., "A Tri-Institutional Approach to Address Disparities in Children's Oncology Group Clinical Trial Accrual for Adolescents and Young Adults and Underrepresented Minorities.", *Journal of Adolescent and Young Adult Oncology*, vol. 8, no. 3 (2019).

[53] Bierer et al., Achieving Diversity.

[54] The Yale Center for Clinical Investigator Cultural Ambassador Program involves partnerships with Junta for Progressive Action—a organization dedicated serving the Hispanic

Ambassadors help promote the Center's clinical trials in the community and work with Center trial staff to create culturally tailored clinical trials information, among other things. Center officials told us that the proportion of patients from diverse backgrounds in clinical trials has increased since implementing the ambassador program in 2010. Specifically, officials reported the proportion of patients in trials from a racial and ethnic group other than non-Hispanic White increased from 3 percent in 2010 to 32 percent in 2021.

- The Fox Chase Cancer Center developed a 7-week community ambassador program to train individuals from Black communities to increase their knowledge of clinical trials and help them feel comfortable discussing clinical trials in the community. The program includes training from Center staff on the history of clinical trials, barriers to participation, and the clinical trial process, including processes to protect patients enrolled in clinical trials. Ambassadors then disseminate clinical trial information within their networks and at community education events, according to officials.

Community advisors. Eleven of the 17 selected cancer centers noted working with community advisors to help them understand the needs of diverse communities within their service area. This is intended to help cancer centers prioritize and design clinical trials to meet the needs of the communities they serve, and help them increase access to trials.

Additionally, we found that three cancer centers noted working with community advisors to develop targeted strategies to engage diverse communities within their service area. Examples of community advisors at the selected cancer centers include the following:

- The University of California Davis Comprehensive Cancer Center community advisory board includes cancer survivors and community members representing rural and urban counties across its service area, as well as community leaders representing racially and ethnically diverse communities. Center staff worked with the community advisory board to help enroll 20 patients from diverse backgrounds in

---

community in greater New Haven—the Connecticut African Methodist Episcopal Zion Churches—one of the oldest Black congregations in the United States, and other community leaders.

a clinical trial for a new device. Board members provided suggestions to make advertisements for the trial more diverse, such as including images of individuals from diverse backgrounds in promotional videos. Center officials said that this input helped them more effectively enroll individuals from diverse backgrounds. The trial received more than 155 inquiries to fill 20 slots, helping them meet their diversity goals.[55]

- The Meharry Medical College, Vanderbilt-Ingram Cancer Center, and Tennessee State University Cancer Partnership has worked with its community advisory board—which includes members from diverse racial and ethnic backgrounds who are cancer survivors, caregivers, and representatives of cancer-related organizations—to facilitate community input into its work. For example, the board developed materials for a clinical trial designed to reduce smoking-related cancer mortalities among racial and ethnic groups other than non-Hispanic White. Board members recommended changes to simplify the language used to describe the interventions to which patients may be assigned. Additionally, board members provided input regarding the tone of the language used to describe trial procedures and enhanced the design of trial materials in a culturally sensitive manner, according to an article describing the Partnership's work with the board.[56]

Workforce-Level Practices

We found that 13 of the 17 selected cancer centers we reviewed noted implementing practices focused on developing an inclusive and diverse health care workforce.[57] These practices include training for health care workers related to the inclusion of patients from diverse backgrounds in clinical trials and efforts to increase diversity within the cancer centers' workforce.

---

[55] R. Badawi et al., "Diversifying the Subject Cohorts in Total-Body PET Research: A Feasibility Study," *Journal of Nuclear Medicine*, vol. 63, no. S2 (2022).

[56] E. Connors et al., "Improving Community Advisory Board Engagement In Precision Medicine Research To Reduce Health Disparities.", *Journal of Health Disparities Research and Practice*, vol. 12: no. 6 (2018).

[57] For the purposes of this report, the "health care workforce" includes both health care providers who provide cancer care, such as physicians and nurses, as well as clinical researchers and research team members, such as those who work on clinical trials.

Workforce training. Nine of the 17 selected cancer centers noted having training for health care workers related to the inclusion of patients from diverse backgrounds in clinical trials. Training in cultural competency— the ability to understand, interact, and work well with people of different cultures—can help health care workers better communicate with diverse patients to increase their awareness of clinical trials.[58] Additionally, training may help health care workers address unconscious biases— attitudes or stereotypes about race, ethnicity, socioeconomic status, or other patient characteristics that unknowingly alter an individuals' perceptions, behavior interactions, and decision-making—that can otherwise lead to inequitable access to trials.[59] Examples of workforce training at the selected cancer centers include the following:

- Duke Cancer Institute's "Just Ask" training program is designed to help health care workers and research teams communicate with patients from diverse backgrounds and ensure patients are aware and knowledgeable about research and clinical trial participation. The program helps workers recognize their own biases and also teaches strategies to mitigate the effects of unconscious biases on the patient experience and clinical trial participation, according to Institute officials. The American Society of Clinical Oncology and the Association of Community Cancer Centers have developed an unconscious bias training based on the Just Ask program that health care workers and research teams from other cancer centers can access online and complete independently.
- The Henry Ford Cancer Institute is developing unconscious bias training for its health care workforce. According to Institute officials, the goal of this training is to increase awareness about the effect of implicit biases on cancer disparities, including to improve clinical trial enrollment among diverse populations.

Diverse health care workforce. Eleven of the 17 selected cancer centers noted implementing practices focused on developing a diverse health care

---

[58] Bierer et al., Achieving Diversity.

[59] N. Barrett et al., "Assessing Feasibility and Utility of an Implicit Bias Training Program for Addressing Disparities in Cancer Clinical Trial Participation." *Journal of Clinical Oncology*, vol. 40, no. 16 (2022).

workforce.[60] A health care workforce that shares the demographic and other characteristics of the diverse communities in their geographic area has been shown to increase participation in clinical research, according to one report.[61] Another report suggested that a diverse health care workforce may help cancer centers increase trust among underrepresented communities.[62] Additionally, a diverse health care workforce can help ensure that clinical trials are designed and implemented to meet the needs of diverse communities, according to a joint statement issued by the American Society of Clinical Oncology and Association of Community Cancer Centers.[63] Examples of efforts to diversify the health care workforce by the selected cancer centers include the following:

- The Henry Ford Cancer Institute established a diversity, equity, inclusion, and justice committee made up of team members across the Institute. The group works to increase awareness and educational opportunities for the Institute's leadership and staff, such as through quarterly learning sessions. It is also focused on increasing diversity in its team members, for example, by working with students from underrepresented backgrounds to increase diversity in the field. The committee reviews the applicant pool to monitor the diversity of candidates and approves all hiring offers before they are made.
- Institute officials noted that hiring individuals from diverse backgrounds who reflect the diversity of communities in the Institute's service area has helped ensure its priorities incorporate the values and needs of all patients.
- The Hollings Cancer Center provides cancer research training and mentoring for students, with a focus on developing the careers of individuals from underrepresented backgrounds. For instance, the Center offers a 10-week summer research program for undergraduate students from three Historically Black Colleges and Universities in South Carolina, as well as the University of South Carolina. The

---

60 For the purpose of this report, a "diverse health care workforce" refers to a workforce that includes individuals from backgrounds identified as underrepresented in the workforce, such women and racial and ethnic groups other than non-Hispanic White, or a workforce that shares the demographic and other characteristics of diverse communities in their geographic area.

61 Bierer et al., *Achieving Diversity*.

62 Garrick et al., "Advancing Inclusive Research".

63 R. A. Oyer et al., "Increasing Racial and Ethnic Diversity in Cancer Clinical Trials: An American Society of Clinical Oncology and Association of Community Cancer Centers Joint Research Statement." *Journal of Clinical Oncology* (2022).

program includes career mentoring from the Center's staff as well as hands-on laboratory research training. Since 2007, many of the students have been included as co-authors on peer-reviewed manuscripts.

Patient-Level Practices Implemented

We found that 15 of the 17 selected cancer centers we reviewed noted implementing practices that are designed to help patients overcome some of the barriers to clinical trial participation. These practices include educating patients about clinical trials, providing culturally and linguistically tailored information, using patient navigators, and providing financial and logistical supports.

Clinical trial education. Fourteen of the 17 selected cancer centers noted implementing practices to help educate patients about clinical trials. This includes practices that are intended to raise patient awareness of trials and trial opportunities, or help patients make informed decisions regarding clinical trial participation. Additionally, one of the centers noted providing clinical trial education to help address mistrust in medical research stemming from a history of racism and research misconduct—a reported barrier to enrolling patients from diverse backgrounds into clinical trials. Examples of clinical trial education for patients at the selected cancer centers include the following:

- Hollings Cancer Center's patient clinical trial education program—the "MOVENUP Train the Trainer Cancer Education Program"—discusses the importance of including diverse populations in cancer clinical trials and includes a focus on addressing mistrust of clinical trials among patients from diverse backgrounds. The program acknowledges previous research misconduct, such as the Tuskegee Study, and then discusses the safeguards that have since been established to protect the rights of clinical trial participants.[64]

---

[64] The Syphilis Study at the Tuskegee Institute, known officially as the "Tuskegee Study of Untreated Syphilis in the Negro Male," was a clinical study run by the U.S. Public Health Service designed to determine the natural course of untreated syphilis in Black men. The study, which ran from 1932 to 1972, followed 600 Black men in Alabama. Researchers did not obtain the patients' consent and told the men they were being treated for "bad blood," a term used to describe several ailments, including syphilis, anemia, and fatigue. Additionally, when penicillin became the standard treatment for the disease in 1943 the medicine was withheld from the patients.

- Fox Chase Cancer Center researchers developed an interactive tool called mychoice that is designed to address racial and ethnic inclusion in medical research. This web-based tool educates patients on clinical trials to help address their concerns related to participation, according to Center officials. As part of mychoice, patients can watch video interviews of cancer patients who have made decisions about participating in clinical trials to hear the concerns these patients had and their approach to deciding whether to participate. Additionally, mychoice provides a list of questions related to clinical trial processes and participation that patients can use to help facilitate discussions with their health care provider. The Center developed mychoice after finding that a lack of information about clinical trials was a barrier to participation for many of their Black patients.

Culturally and linguistically tailored information. Ten of the 17 selected cancer centers noted having clinical trial information that is tailored to meet the needs of culturally and linguistically diverse patients. To help people make informed decisions about trial participation, study materials must be culturally, linguistically, and ethnically appropriate, according a joint statement issued by the American Society of Clinical Oncology and Association of Community Cancer Centers.[65] We found that six centers have also used culturally and linguistically tailored information to help increase patient trust, awareness, and knowledge of trials. Examples of culturally and linguistically tailored information at the selected cancer centers include the following:

- The University of California Davis Comprehensive Cancer Center offers clinical trial education materials in English, as well as Hmong, Vietnamese, Cantonese, Mandarin, and Korean—languages the Center identified through a community needs assessment on clinical trial knowledge. Providing materials in a patient's native language helps to increase trust and education among individuals with limited English proficiency, and has played a critical role in the enrollment of Asian American cancer patients into clinical trials, according to Center officials. Additionally, Center officials reported that the center has translated research materials, such as information sheets and patient consent forms, into Spanish. These materials were reviewed

[65] Oyer et al., "Increasing Racial and Ethnic Diversity in Cancer Clinical Trials".

by six bilingual and bicultural staff to ensure correct translation and that the materials are culturally appropriate for the Latino community, according to Center officials.

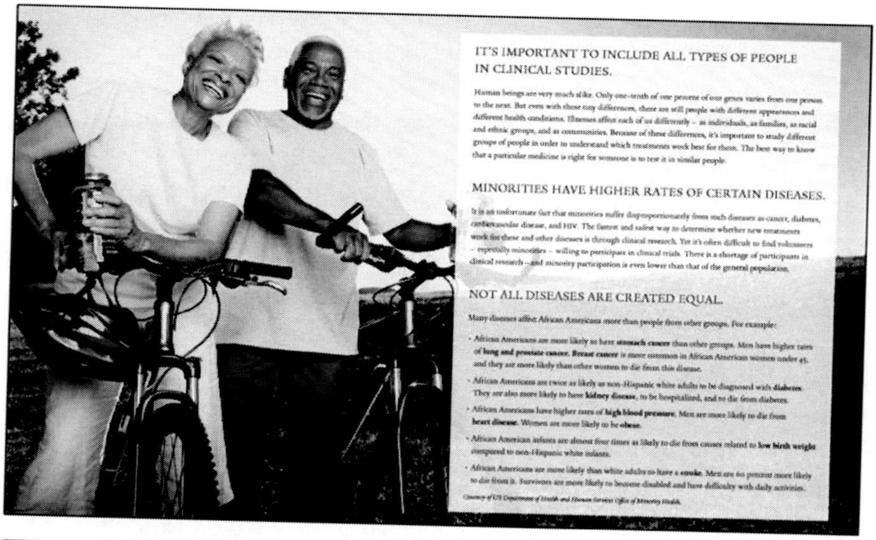
IT'S IMPORTANT TO INCLUDE ALL TYPES OF PEOPLE IN CLINICAL STUDIES.
MINORITIES HAVE HIGHER RATES OF CERTAIN DISEASES.
NOT ALL DISEASES ARE CREATED EQUAL.

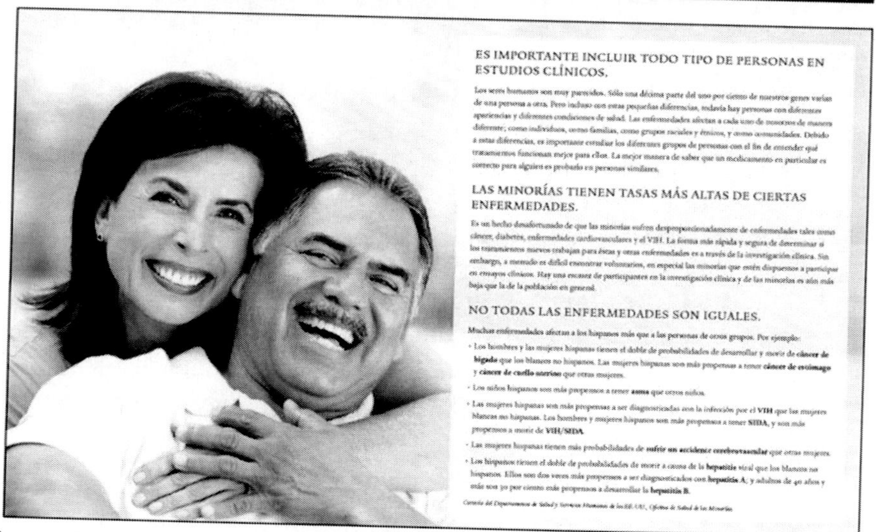
ES IMPORTANTE INCLUIR TODO TIPO DE PERSONAS EN ESTUDIOS CLÍNICOS.
LAS MINORÍAS TIENEN TASAS MÁS ALTAS DE CIERTAS ENFERMEDADES.
NO TODAS LAS ENFERMEDADES SON IGUALES.

Source: Yale Center for Clinical Investigation. | GAO-23-105245.

Figure 4. Yale Clinical Trial Education Materials for Black and Hispanic Patients.

- As part of its "Help Us Discover" clinical trial awareness campaign, the Yale Center for Clinical Investigation developed culturally and linguistically tailored advertisements and education to promote its clinical research and encourage diverse participation. Specifically, the Center created education brochures that included photos of Black and Hispanic individuals and information describing why diverse representation in clinical trials is important. Additionally, the brochure was available in Spanish. (See fig. 4.)

Patient navigators. Ten of the 17 selected cancer centers noted having patient navigators—center staff or lay health workers responsible for guiding a patient through the healthcare system—to support patients and educate them on clinical trials. Research suggests that patient navigators may help cancer centers enroll diverse patients in clinical trials by providing practical support that enhances initial enrollment and continued support for participants enrolled in trials to enhance retention.[66] For instance, one report found that patient navigators can help identify whether there are barriers to patients' participation in a clinical trial and assist them in addressing those barriers, such as by helping with manage transportation and lodging.[67] Additionally, by educating patients on trials, patient navigators can raise awareness of trials and help ensure patients have the information they need to make informed decisions regarding clinical trial participation.

- One example of this is Avera Health's "Walking Forward" program, which includes two types of patient navigators—navigators who are based at the Center in Rapid City, and lay navigators who are members of American Indian communities. Navigators based in the Center assist American Indian patients with coordinating appointments, insurance issues, following up on tests, obtaining medications and specialty services or devices, facilitating transportation and lodging, and offer psychosocial support during treatment. Lay navigators work closely with the hospital staff and educate cancer patients on clinical trials, access to cancer screening and enrollment in community trials such as lung cancer screening and palliative care projects.

---

66 K. B. Cartmell et al., "Patient Barriers to Cancer Clinical Trial Participation and Navigator Activities." *Advances in Cancer Research*, vol. 146 (2020); M. N. Fouad et al., "Patient Navigation as a Model to Increase Participation of African Americans in Cancer Clinical Trials." *Journal of Oncology Practice*, vol. 12, no. 6 (2016).

67 K. B. Cartmell et al, "Patient Barriers and Navigator Activities".

Financial and logistical support. Eight of the 17 selected cancer centers noted providing financial or logistical support for patients enrolled in trials. This may help cancer centers enroll patients from diverse backgrounds, as research suggests that patients from diverse backgrounds are more likely to be underrepresented in cancer clinical trials due to limited financial resources.[68] Logistical issues, such as having to take time off work and needing to find transportation to and from the trial site, can also be a barrier. Examples of financial and logistical support provided at the selected cancer centers include the following:

- Duke Cancer Institute patients, including those enrolled in clinical trials, who meet financial eligibility guidelines may receive support for out-of-pocket expenses, including transportation and lodging, according to Institute officials. Patients may also receive lodging through community partners such as Caring House, a non-profit organization that provides supportive and affordable housing to patients.
- Henry Ford Cancer Institute officials reported that the Institute uses its "Game On Cancer" campaign to support cancer patients. The campaign—a partnership between Henry Ford and the Detroit Lions football team, the Detroit Pistons basketball team, and other corporate partners—raises funds through special events to support patients and clinical research. According to Institute officials, this effort helps alleviate financial challenges cancer patients and their families may experience by providing the funds to pay for transportation, housing, prescriptions, medical supplies, and other expenses. Since the campaign started in 2015, Game On Cancer has raised more than $5 million, according to officials.

Agency Comments

We provided a draft of this report to DOD, HHS, and VA for review. The agencies provided technical comments, which we incorporated as appropriate.

We are sending copies of this report to the appropriate congressional committees, the Secretary of Defense, the Secretary of Health and Human Services, the Secretary of Veterans Affairs, and other interested parties. In

[68] R. D. Nipp et al., "Addressing the Financial Burden".

addition, the report is available at no charge on the GAO website at https://www.gao.gov.

If you or your staff have any questions about this report, please contact me at (202) 512-7114 or DickenJ@gao.gov. Contact points for our Offices of Congressional Relations and Public Affairs may be found on the last page of this report. GAO staff who made key contributions to this report are listed in appendix IV.

John E. Dicken
Director, Health Care

List of Committees

The Honorable Patty Murray
Chair

The Honorable Richard Burr
Ranking Member
Committee on Health, Education, Labor and Pensions
United States Senate

The Honorable Patty Murray
Chair

The Honorable Roy Blunt
Ranking Member
Subcommittee on Labor, Health and Human Services,
Education and Related Agencies Committee on Appropriations
United States Senate

The Honorable Frank Pallone, Jr.
Chairman

The Honorable Cathy McMorris Rodgers
Republican Leader
Committee on Energy and Commerce
House of Representatives

The Honorable Rosa DeLauro
Chair
The Honorable Tom Cole
Ranking Member
Subcommittee on Labor, Health and Human Services,
Education and Related Agencies Committee on Appropriations
House of Representatives

Appendix I: Objectives, Scope, and Methodology

Our report examined the following: (1) actions federal agencies have taken to facilitate enrollment of patients from diverse backgrounds in cancer clinical trials and (2) practices used by selected cancer centers to facilitate enrollment of patients from diverse backgrounds in cancer clinical trials. For the purposes of this report, we focused on diversity in terms of racial and ethnic groups, adolescents and young adults, older adults, women, low-income individuals, and individuals from rural communities because they were either specified in the legislation or had been cited in scientific literature as underrepresented groups in clinical trials. We used the National Cancer Institute's definition of clinical trials, which includes those studies to test new methods of screening, prevention, diagnosis, or treatment. We use the word "centers" to describe cancer centers and institutes.

To address our research objectives, we

1. interviewed federal officials and stakeholders representing patient advocacy groups, pharmaceutical companies, and clinical research professionals and organizations;
2. reviewed relevant guidance and documents from federal officials;
3. conducted a review of relevant literature and publicly available information to identify cancer centers that enrolled a larger than average proportion of patients from diverse backgrounds in cancer clinical trials or been recognized in published literature for doing so; and

4. analyzed responses from questionnaires provided to selected cancer centers to identify the practices they have implemented.

We conducted this performance audit from May 2021 to December 2022 in accordance with generally accepted government auditing standards. Those standards require that we plan and perform the audit to obtain sufficient, appropriate evidence to provide a reasonable basis for our findings and conclusions based on our audit objectives. We believe that the evidence obtained provides a reasonable basis for our findings and conclusions based on our audit objectives.

Interviews with Federal Officials and Stakeholders

To address both objectives, we conducted semi-structured interviews with numerous federal officials and stakeholders who could provide a variety of perspectives on issues related to diversity in cancer clinical trials,

- The Department of Health and Human Services (HHS), including the Food and Drug Administration (FDA), the National Institutes of Health (NIH), the Centers for Disease Control and Prevention, the Office of Minority Health, and the Centers for Medicare & Medicaid Services (CMS);
- The Department of Veterans Affairs (VA), including Veterans Health Administration; and
- The Department of Defense (DOD), including the Congressionally Directed Medical Research Programs (CDMRP) and Murtha Cancer Center.

We also interviewed 13 stakeholders that represent a variety of perspectives in patient advocacy, clinical research, and the pharmaceutical industry. These stakeholders provided various perspectives on the issues under study, as well as information about potential cancer centers to include in our review. We identified potential stakeholders—organizations or individual experts— through literature on clinical trials, as well as through our interviews. We identified those that had a history of focusing on both cancer and clinical trials and conducted interviews with the following:

- Patient advocates: American Cancer Society Cancer Action Network; Friends of Cancer Research; National Minority Quality Forum; and a long-time health advocate.
- Clinical research organizations: American Society of Clinical Oncology; Association of Community Cancer Centers; the Patient-Centered Outcomes Research Institute, an independent, non-profit, non-federal organization authorized by the Patient Protection and Affordable Care Act; and the Society of Gynecologic Oncology.
- Clinical researchers: A Bloomberg Distinguished Professor at the John Hopkins University who is an expert in cancer prevention and control; and an Associate Professor in the Cancer Prevention Program at the Fred Hutchinson Cancer Center and Assistant Professor at the University of Washington School of Public Health, with a background in health services research who focuses on cancer outcomes and disparities.
- Pharmaceutical industry representatives: Eli Lilly and Company, Genentech, and the Pharmaceutical Research and Manufacturers of America, which represents pharmaceutical and biotechnology companies.

Review of Federal Actions, Policies and Guidance, and Practices

To describe the actions federal agencies have taken to include diverse representation in cancer clinical trial participation, we analyzed interviews we conducted with federal officials from the agencies named above as well as additional information about the actions as reported on agency websites. We also reviewed and analyzed documents from the federal agencies that outline relevant agency policies (including guidance) and practices related to clinical trial participation. A complete list of federal guidance we reviewed is in app. II.

Identification of Selected Cancer Centers and Their Practices

To describe practices that facilitate diverse representation in cancer clinical trial participation, we identified non-federal cancer centers that enrolled a larger than average proportion of patients from diverse backgrounds in cancer clinical trials or were recognized in academic journals for doing so. We then fielded a questionnaire to these centers to learn more about the practices that they have implemented.

Identification of Selected Cancer Centers

To identify those cancer centers that enrolled patients from diverse backgrounds, we asked federal officials and stakeholders to identify such centers directly or for articles that described such centers. For example, one article described eight cancer centers that had sustained participation of ethnic minorities between 10 percent and 50 percent per trial.[69]

We also conducted a literature search to identify cancer centers. We searched SCOPUS, PubMed, and all available collections in ProQuest, EBSCO, and Dialog databases for materials published since 2017 that identified or described cancer centers that enroll underrepresented populations.[70] From this search, we identified 38 unique and potentially relevant articles. We reviewed each article to determine if it focused on diverse representation in cancer clinical trials, versus clinical trials more broadly, and the inclusion of the underrepresented groups cited above.[71] For each article that met this criteria, we further reviewed the article to determine if it described activities that were in operation during the prior 5 years. We also looked for evidence of effectiveness in enrolling patients of diverse backgrounds. One way to demonstrate this was through data showing that the center enrolled high numbers of underrepresented groups or has increased the participation of underrepresented groups since implementing practices to increase diverse representation. Another way was external recognition of the

---

69 J. M. Regnante, et al., "US Cancer Centers of Excellence Strategies for Increased Inclusion of Racial and Ethnic Minorities in Clinical Trials." *Journal of Oncology Practice,* vol. 15, no. 4 (2019).

70 The search terms we used were cancer clinical trials; oncology clinical trials; exemplary programs, promising programs, notable programs, programs of excellence (and programs can be "programs", "practices" or "centers"); enrollment, accrual, recruitment, retention; minorities; racial diversity; representation, underrepresentation; community outreach, community engagement, community partnership; community advisory board; peer support, patient navigators, lay navigators, community ambassadors; provider education and training; cultural competence, cultural awareness; culturally sensitive recruitment; mobile clinics; and telehealth.

71 The centers may serve other populations not in the scope of how we define diversity for purposes of this report.

center as enrolling diverse populations. Of the 38 articles, four met this criteria.[72]

Based on these combined efforts, we identified 17 cancer centers for our review. Because our selection methodology was not exhaustive, there may be other centers we did not identify that also enrolled diverse populations into cancer clinical trials. The selected cancer centers we identified were the following:

- Abramson Cancer Center
- Avera Health
- Benefis Sletten Cancer Institute
- Children's Oncology Group – University of Illinois at Chicago, Rush University Medical Center, and John H. Stroger Hospital
- Duke Cancer Institute
- Fox Chase Cancer Center
- Harold C. Simmons Comprehensive Cancer Center
- Henry Ford Cancer Institute
- Hollings Cancer Center
- Mary Bird Perkins Cancer Center
- Meharry Medical College, Vanderbilt-Ingram Cancer Center, and Tennessee State University Cancer Partnership
- University of California at Davis Comprehensive Cancer Center
- University of New Mexico Cancer Research and Treatment Center
- University of Texas MD Anderson Cancer Center
- Winship Cancer Institute
- Yale Cancer Center and Yale Center for Clinical Investigation
- Yuma Regional Medical Center Cancer Center

[72] J. M. Regnante et al., "Abstract PO-096: A Guide for Development of a Successful and Inclusive Lung Cancer Research Strategy Based on U.S. Best Practices." *Cancer Epidemiology Biomarkers Prevention, vol. 29, no. 12* (2020); J. M. Regnante, et al., "Operational Strategies in US Cancer Centers of Excellence that Support the Successful Accrual of Racial and Ethnic Minorities in Clinical Trials." *Contemporary Clinical Trials Communications*, vol. 17 (2020); A. Trant et al., "Increasing Accrual of Minority Patients in Breast Cancer Clinical Trials." *Breast Cancer Research and Treatment,* vol. 184 (2020); N. Mittal et al., "A Tri-Institutional Approach to Address Disparities in Children's Oncology Group Clinical Trial Accrual for Adolescents and Young Adults and Underrepresented Minorities.", *Journal of Adolescent and Young Adult Oncology*, vol. 8, no. 3 (2019).

Identification of Practices

To identify examples of practices—the activities each of these cancer centers uses to facilitate enrollment of patients from diverse backgrounds in cancer clinical trials—we asked representatives from each of the selected cancer centers to complete a written questionnaire we developed. We sent the questionnaire via email in March and April 2022. The first part of the questionnaire asked about the specific activities the center has used or uses to facilitate the recruitment and retention of patients from diverse backgrounds in cancer trials. We prefilled the questionnaire with the activities we were already aware of from the literature and asked the center to make corrections or add any we may have missed. For each of the activities, the questionnaire asked the center officials to provide supporting documentation where available. The second part of the questionnaire asked more general questions about the center as a whole, such as examples of notable practices, populations of interest, and how the center's activities function together.

Of the 17 centers we asked to complete our questionnaire, 13 (76 percent) returned completed questionnaires by May 2022. We then analyzed the responses to develop categories of activities that the cancer centers described.[73] We included examples of these activities in the report. For those four cancer centers that did not return the questionnaire, we used publicly available information to describe their activities. We provided representatives of the 13 centers that completed the questionnaire the opportunity to review the parts of the draft report relevant to their center and incorporated technical comments, as appropriate. We did not independently verify the information reported by the centers in their response to the questionnaires we sent them or from published sources.

Appendix II: Federal Agency Guidance and Policy Related to Diversity in Clinical Trials

Below is a list of guidance and policy documents from the Food and Drug Administration (FDA) and National Institutes of Health (NIH) related to improving diversity in clinical trials, and issued since 2014. Those that are not specific to cancer clinical trials are still relevant to them.

---

[73] We did not evaluate the effectiveness of the specific categories of activities that the cancer centers described.

U. S. Department of Health and Human Services, Food and Drug Administration. *Diversity Plans to Improve Enrollment of Participants from Underrepresented Racial and Ethnic Populations in Clinical Trials – Guidance for Industry* (Draft Guidance). Silver Spring, MD: Apr. 2022.

U. S. Department of Health and Human Services, Food and Drug Administration. *Inclusion of Older Adults in Cancer Clinical Trials – Guidance for Industry*. Silver Spring, MD: Mar. 2022.

U. S. Department of Health and Human Services, Food and Drug Administration. *Digital Health Technologies for Remote Data Acquisition in Clinical Investigation (Draft Guidance for Industry, Investigators, and Other Stakeholders)*. Silver Spring, MD: Jan. 2022.

U. S. Department of Health and Human Services, Food and Drug Administration. *Enhancing the Diversity of Clinical Trial Populations—Eligibility Criteria, Enrollment Practices, and Trial Designs – Guidance for Industry.* Silver Spring, MD: Nov. 2020.

U. S. Department of Health and Human Services, Food and Drug Administration. *Conduct of Clinical Trials of Medical Products during the COVID-19 Public Health Emergency — Guidance for Industry, Investigators, and Institutional Review Boards.* Silver Spring, MD: Mar. 2020, updated Aug. 2021.

U. S. Department of Defense, Department of the Army, *The CDMRP Policy and Guidelines on the Inclusion of Women and Minorities as Subjects in Clinical Research.* Fort Detrick, MD: July 2020.

U. S. Department of Health and Human Services, National Institutes of Health, National Cancer Institute. *Interim Guidance for Patients on Clinical Trials Supported by the NCI Cancer Therapy Evaluation Program and the NCI Community Oncology Research Program (NCORP)*. Bethesda, MD: Mar. 2020.

U. S. Department of Health and Human Services, Food and Drug Administration. *Payment and Reimbursement to Research Subjects - Guidance for Institutional Review Boards and Clinical Investigators* (Information Sheet). Silver Spring, MD: Jan. 2018.

U. S. Department of Health and Human Services, National Institutes of Health. *Revision: NIH Policy and Guidelines on the Inclusion of Individuals across the Lifespan as Participants in Research Involving Human Subjects,* NOT-OD-18-116. Bethesda, MD: Dec. 2017.

U. S. Department of Health and Human Services, National Institutes of Health. *Amendment: NIH Policy and Guidelines on the Inclusion of Women and Minorities as Subjects in Clinical Research,* NOT-OD-18-014. Bethesda, MD: Nov. 2017.

U. S. Department of Health and Human Services, Food and Drug Administration. *Collection of Race and Ethnicity Data in Clinical Trials – Guidance for Industry and Food and Drug Administration Staff.* Silver Spring, MD: Oct. 2016.

U. S. Department of Health and Human Services, Food and Drug Administration. *Action Plan to Enhance the Collection and Availability of Demographic Subgroup Data.* Silver Spring, MD: Aug. 2014.

Appendix III: Selected Cancer Center Practices Related to Diversity in Clinical Trials

The 17 selected cancer centers have implemented various practices to help facilitate the enrollment of patients from diverse backgrounds in cancer clinical trials. Figures 5 through 17 include descriptions of some of the relevant practices from the 13 cancer centers that responded to the questionnaire we sent.

Case Example: Initiative to Enroll Black Patients Into Cancer Clinical Trials

In 2014, Abramson Cancer Center implemented an initiative to increase the enrollment of Black patients into cancer clinical trials. As part of the initiative, the Center promoted clinical trials addressing cancers that affected Black residents and required that each trial have a plan to recruit Black patients. The initiative also included: culturally tailored marketing strategies, community education by faith-based organizations serving Black communities, transportation through ride-sharing companies to and from appointments, and patient education by nurse navigators.

These efforts have reached more than 10,000 individuals and doubled the percentage of Black patients enrolled in the Center's cancer clinical trials. From 2014 through 2018, the percentage of Black patients enrolled in cancer treatment trials increased from 12.2 percent to 23.9 percent.

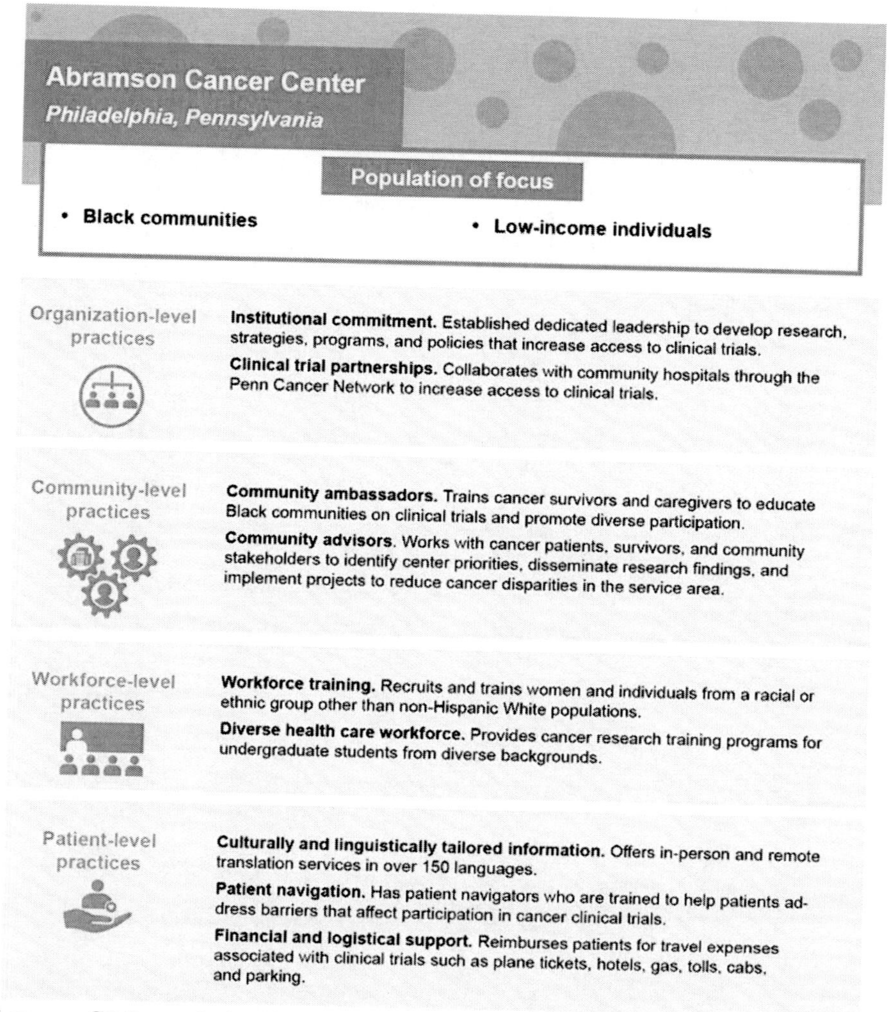

Source: GAO analysis of cancer quiestionnarie responces and other public information. | GAO-23-105245.

Figure 5. Selected Abramson Cancer Center Practices to Facilitate Diverse Patient Representation in Clinical Trials.

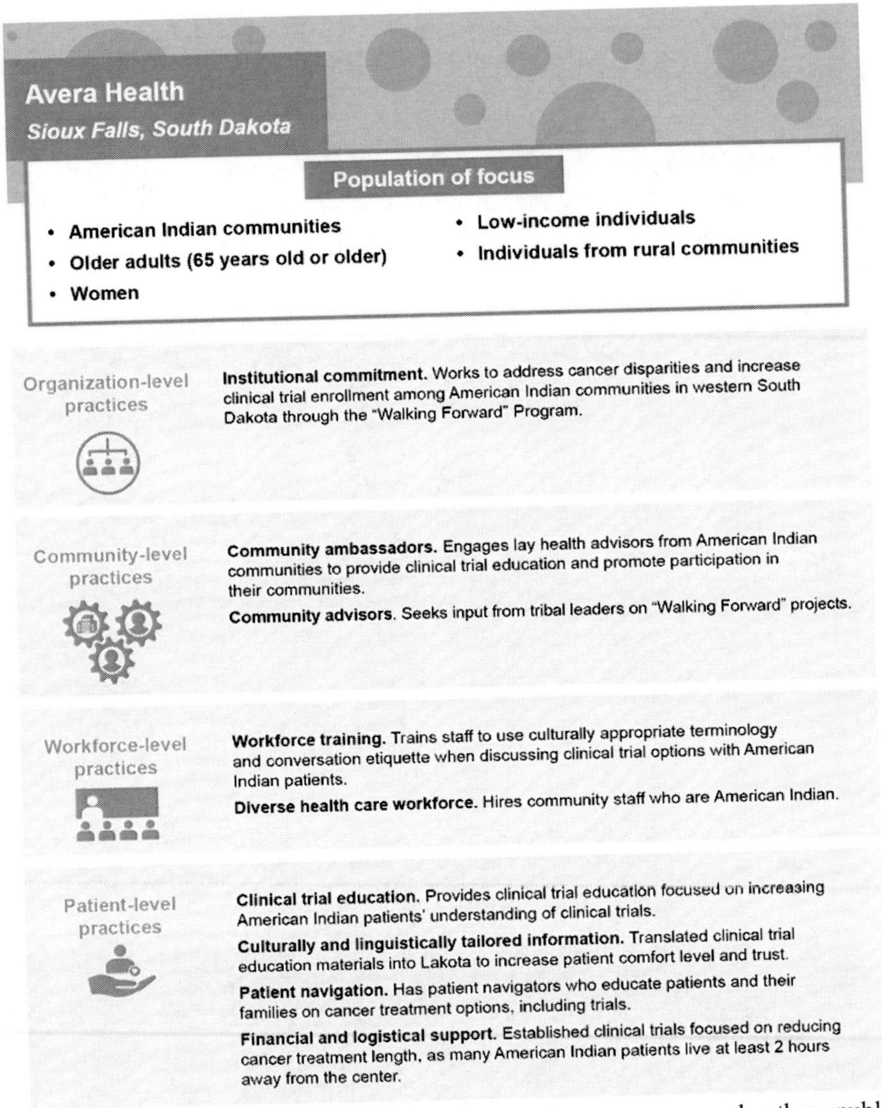

Source: GAO analysis of cancer quiestionnarie responces and other public information. | GAO-23-105245.

Figure 6. Selected Avera Health Practices to Facilitate Diverse Patient Representation in Clinical Trials.

Case example: Program to enroll American Indian patients in cancer clinical trials

Avera Health's "Walking Forward" program is focused on enrolling American Indians in cancer clinical trials to help decrease the high cancer mortality rates among American Indian populations living in western South Dakota—specifically, communities living in Rapid City, South Dakota, and on the Pine Ridge, Rosebud, and Cheyenne River reservations. To increase participation, "Walking Forward" has done the following:

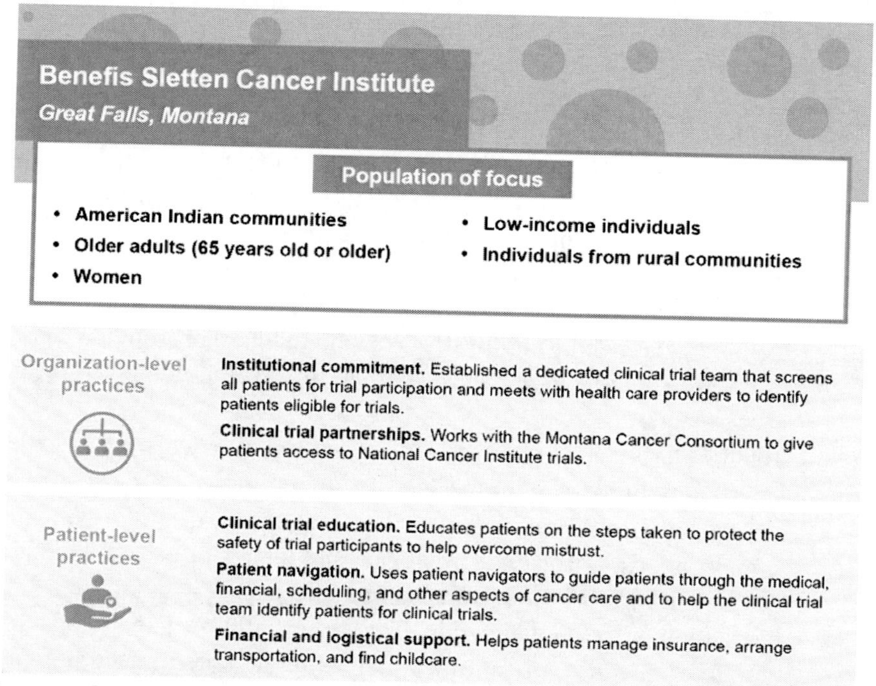

Source: GAO analysis of cancer quiestionnarie responces and other public information. | GAO-23-105245.

Figure 7. Selected Benefis Sletten Cancer Institute Practices to Facilitate Diverse Patient Representation in Clinical Trials.

- Implemented community surveys to evaluate barriers to accessing care.
- Created culturally tailored education on cancer screening and clinical trial opportunities.

- Engaged American Indian patient navigators and community research representatives to increase community trust, improve access to early diagnosis and treatment, and support the needs patients.

Since it was established in 2002, "Walking Forward" has enrolled 4,500 American Indian patients—the highest in the nation, according to program officials.

Case Example: Efforts to Engage Rural and American Indian Communities

Benefis Sletten Cancer Institute provides care to a 13-county region in central Montana. The Center's service area includes rural communities and approximately 20 percent of patients live more than 100 miles from the Center. There are also three reservations and one federally recognized but landless tribe within the Center's service area. About 7 percent of patients are American Indian. To help provide diverse communities access to care and clinical trials, Center offers the following:

- Complementary housing for patients who live farther from the center to relieve some of the financial burden of traveling to and from the cancer center.
- Telehealth services so that patients can receive care when travel to the Center is not possible, for instance due to weather.
- A Welcoming Center that provides culturally sensitive care and support for American Indian patients and their families, including a cultural room for smudging ceremonies and a quiet area for meditation or traditional prayer. This helps build trust and allows for continued practice of spiritual and cultural beliefs, according to Center officials.

The Center has between 80 and 120 trials open for enrollment, and about 4 percent of its patients are enrolled in clinical trials annually.

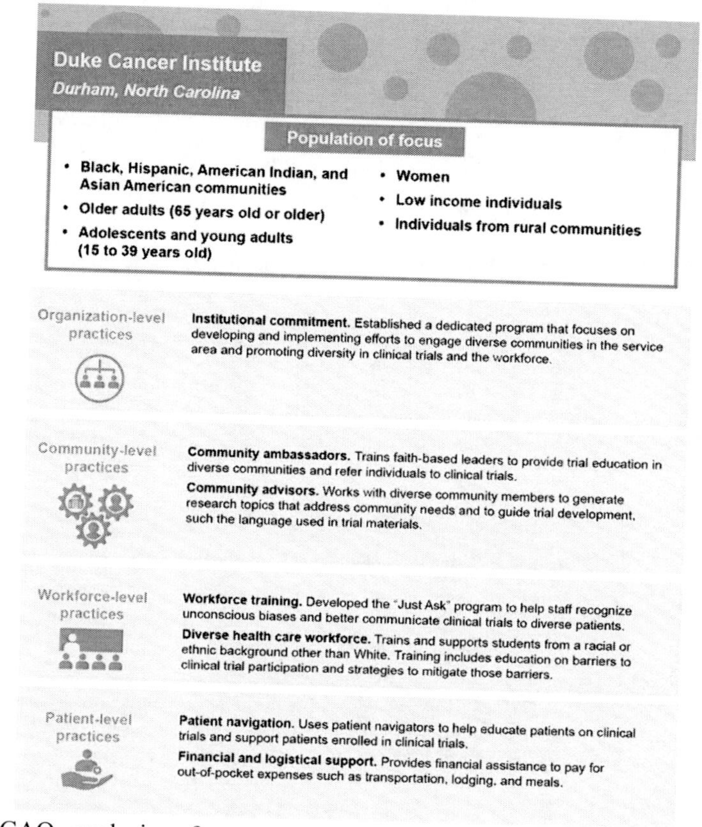

Source: GAO analysis of cancer quiestionnarie responces and other public information. | GAO-23-105245.

Figure 8. Selected Duke Cancer institute Practices to Facilitate Diverse Patient Representation in Clinical Trials.

Case Example: Training the Health Care Workforce

The Duke Cancer Institute provides training on diversity and inclusion in the workforce and clinical trials for staff and for students from diverse backgrounds to increase retention in the academic pipeline. For example, the Institute has implemented the following programs:

- The "Just Ask" training program helps staff recognize unconscious biases and teaches them strategies to mitigate the effect of unconscious biases on the participation of patients from diverse backgrounds in clinical trials.

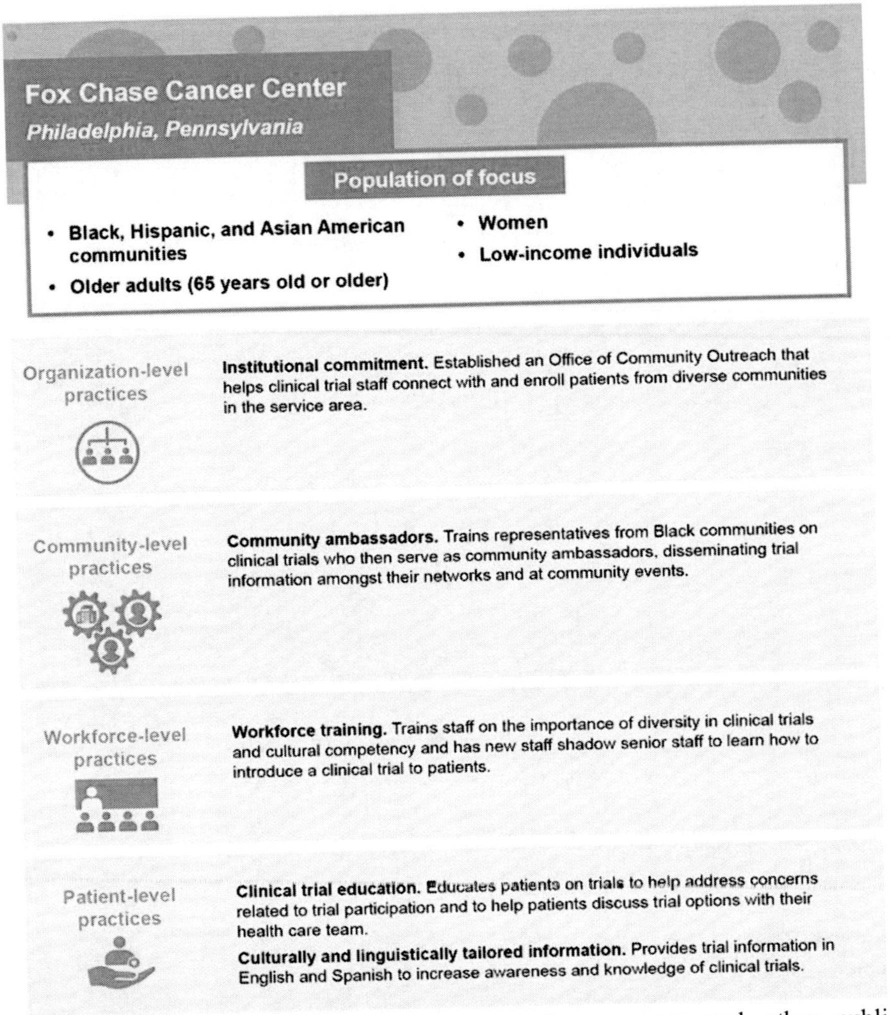

Source: GAO analysis of cancer quiestionnarie responces and other public information. | GAO-23-105245.

Figure 9. Selected Fox Chase Cancer Center Practices to Facilitate Diverse Patient Representation in Clinical Trials.

- The "Cancer Research Education Program" trains students from diverse backgrounds at Duke and North Carolina Central University, a historically black university, to improve their skills in recognizing biases and addressing issues of equity and inclusion within professional settings. The program also includes training on community engagement, barriers to enrolling diverse patients in clinical trials, and strategies to help address enrollment barriers.

- According to Center officials, the "Diversifying Research and Experiential Learning in Cancer Training Fellowship" program promotes cancer research equity among trainees from diverse backgrounds through mentorship, professional development, and science communication.
- A five-part training program educates and mobilizes health care workers and scientists on strategies for community engagement, according to Center officials.

Case Example: Efforts to Educate Patients on Clinical Trials

The Fox Chase Cancer Center is focused on increasing clinical trial awareness and knowledge among diverse communities and patients from diverse backgrounds to help enrollment in clinical trials. The Center has worked to developed several efforts to support this goal:

- The "Be the Breakthrough" campaign provides patients with clinical trial information in English and Spanish to encourage patients to discuss clinical trial options with their health care provider.
- The Preparatory Education About Clinical Trials education program provides general information about clinical trials to help patients better understand what trials are and how they work. Information is provided through a series of short videos.
- Mychoice is a web-based education tool that was designed to address concerns related to clinical trial participation and to help patients facilitate conversations about clinical trials with their health care providers. The tool has been adapted to reflect multi-cultural audiences and, according to Center officials, will be available in multiple languages.
- The Community Bilingual Speakers Bureau provides cancer education on a variety of cancer topics including: breast, cervical, colorectal, liver, lung, ovarian, prostate and skin. All topics provide an overview of what cancer is, risk factors, symptoms, screening guidelines, and treatment option including clinical trials.

Case Example: Project to The Enrollment of Black Patients in Cancer Clinical Trials

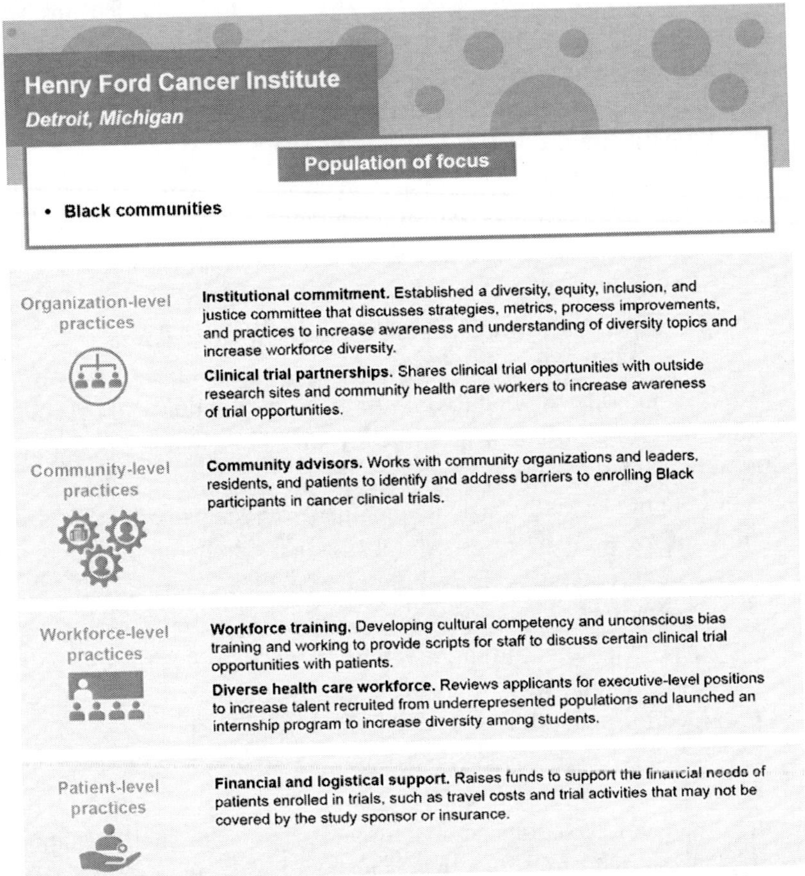

Source: GAO analysis of cancer quiestionnarie responces and other public information. | GAO-23-105245.

Figure 10. Selected Henry Ford Cancer Institute Practices to Facilitate Diverse Patient Representation in Clinical Trials.

In 2021, the Henry Ford Cancer Institute initiated the Participatory Action for Access to Clinical Trials project with the goal of improving the representation of Black individuals in cancer clinical trials. The Institute conducted focus groups and interviews with patients and survivors, community members, and providers and research staff to better understand barriers to clinical trial participation and Black individuals' attitudes about research. The goal is to use this information to understand whether there are opportunities to better engage Black patients in clinical trials and to develop and test interventions to overcome identified barriers.

The project is being implemented in collaboration with community organizations and leaders and will focus on clinical trials involving breast, colorectal, lung, and prostate cancers, which are more likely to result in death for Black individuals when compared to other racial and ethnic groups.

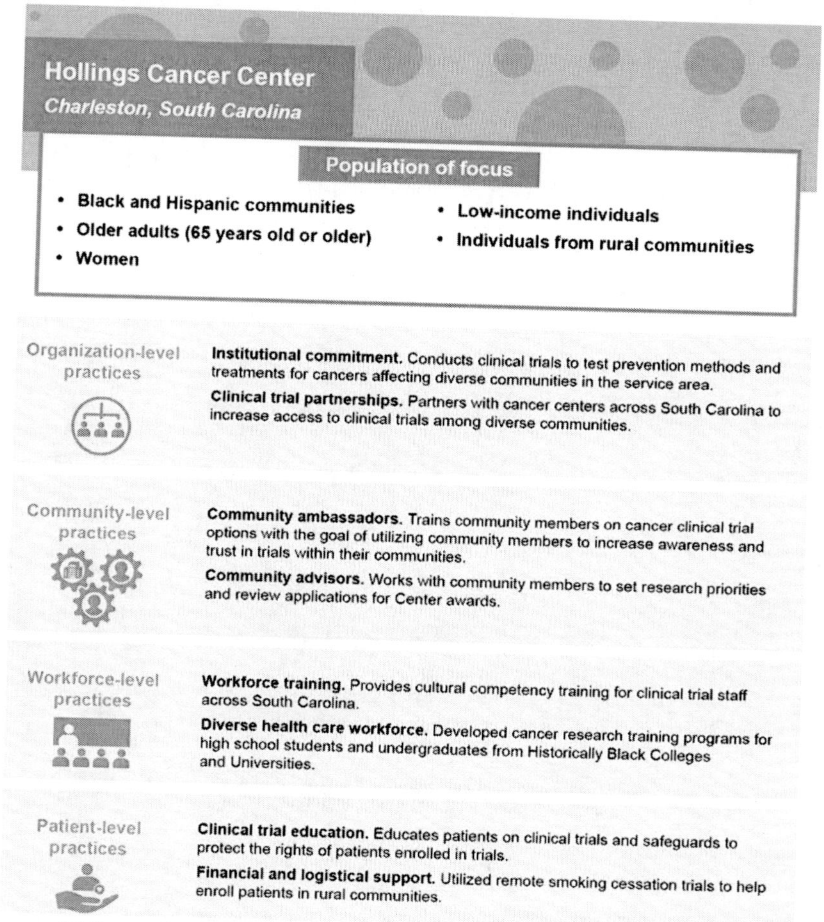

Source: GAO analysis of cancer quiestionnarie responces and other public information. | GAO-23-105245.

Figure 11. Selected Hollings Cancer Center Practices to Facilitate Diverse Patient Representation in Clinical Trials.

Case Example: Program to Address Prostate Cancer Disparities

In September 2021, Hollings Cancer Center initiated a 3-year program to reduce prostate cancer disparities in its service area by increasing prostate cancer screening rates among Black men aged 40 to 69 in South Carolina. Prostate cancer is the second leading cause of cancer death among Black men in South Carolina, and the mortality rate among Black men with prostate cancer is 2.5 times higher than among White men. To increase screening, Hollings will deliver monthly prostate cancer education sessions and provide navigation services for those who attend education sessions to address barriers they may face in getting prostate cancer screening.

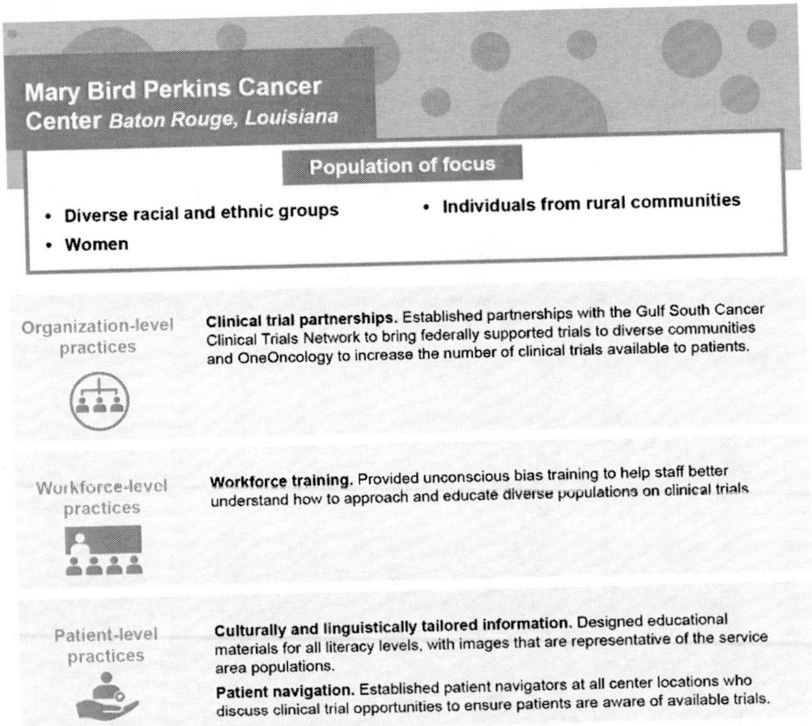

Source: GAO analysis of cancer quiestionnarie responces and other public information. | GAO-23-105245.

Figure 12. Selected Mary Bird Perkins Cancer Center Practices to Facilitate Diverse Patient Representation in Clinical Trials.

As of November 2022, Center officials report that 156 Black men had enrolled in the trial and 93 percent of the men enrolled were navigated to prostate cancer screening or had made an appointment to get screened for prostate cancer. Center officials said they expect the effort will help guide the development and implementation of future trials focused on cancer prevention, control, and treatment strategies for Black men.

Case example: Clinical trial partnerships to expand clinical trial availability

The Mary Bird Cancer Center is an independent, community-owned, nonprofit cancer center that serves diverse communities throughout southeast Louisiana and southwest Mississippi. Four of the six areas in which the Center has a facility have a Black majority population. The Center partners with the Gulf South Minority Underserved NCI Community Oncology Research Program Cancer Clinical Trials Network and OneOncology, which helps the Center meet its goal of offering a number of trial opportunities to patients.

- Participating in the Gulf South Minority Underserved NCI Community Oncology Research Program Cancer Clinical Trials Network enables the Center to offer NCI supported cancer clinical trials to its patients. The network consists of cancer centers and health care providers in Louisiana and Mississippi that work together to improve patient outcomes by expanding access to cancer prevention and treatment trials as well by providing community based outreach and education programs. Collectively, the network offers cancer trials at more than 40 locations.
- In January 2022, the Center established a partnership with OneOncology, a national platform that provides operational, regulatory, and research services for independent cancer practices. The partnership will enable the Center's patients to access clinical trials OneOncology is participating in, offering additional opportunities for them to participate in a study that may enhance their treatment.

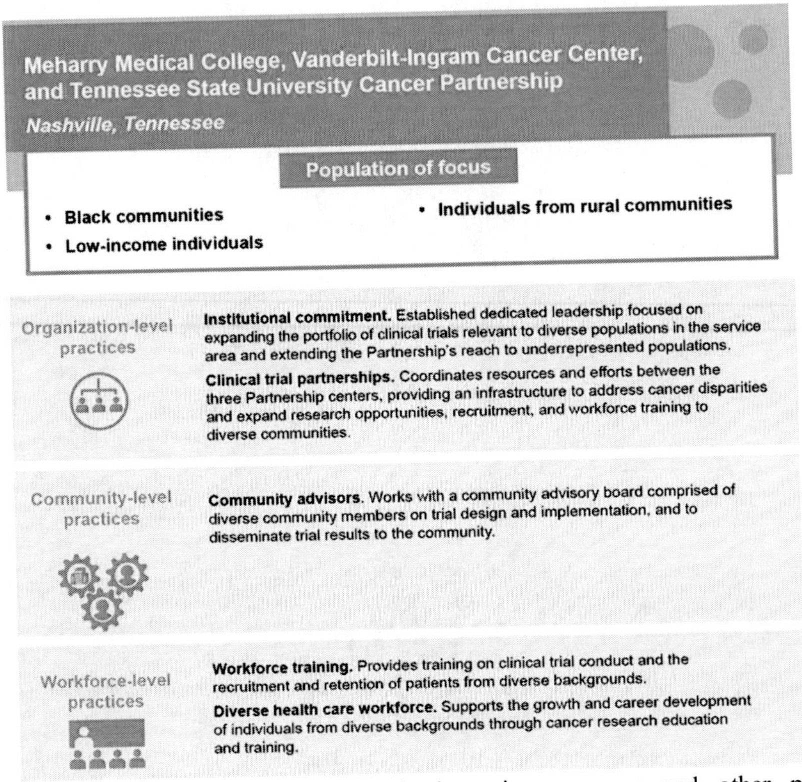

Source: GAO analysis of cancer quiestionnarie responces and other public information. | GAO-23-105245.

Figure 13. Selected Meharry Medical College, Vanderbilt-Ingram Cancer Center, and Tennessee State University Cancer Partnership Practices to Facilitate Diverse Patient Representation in Clinical Trials.

Case Example: Community Engagement and Workforce Training Efforts

The Meharry Medical College, Vanderbilt-Ingram Cancer Center, and Tennessee State Cancer Partnership is a collaboration between three programs in Nashville, Tennessee, focused on increasing the diversity of the health care workforce and the enrollment of patients from diverse backgrounds in cancer clinical trials. The Partnership has developed the dedicated programs to support community outreach and workforce training.

- The cancer outreach program works with community partners to help ensure that the Partnership's activities reflect the needs and concerns of diverse communities in the service area and to provide community-based education. The program also conducts events focused on recruiting and referring Black and Hispanic patients to cancer clinical trials.

- The "Pathway to Discovery" program provides cancer research education for high school students from diverse backgrounds to increase their awareness of careers in cancer research. The program also supports students from Meharry Medical College and Tennessee State University.

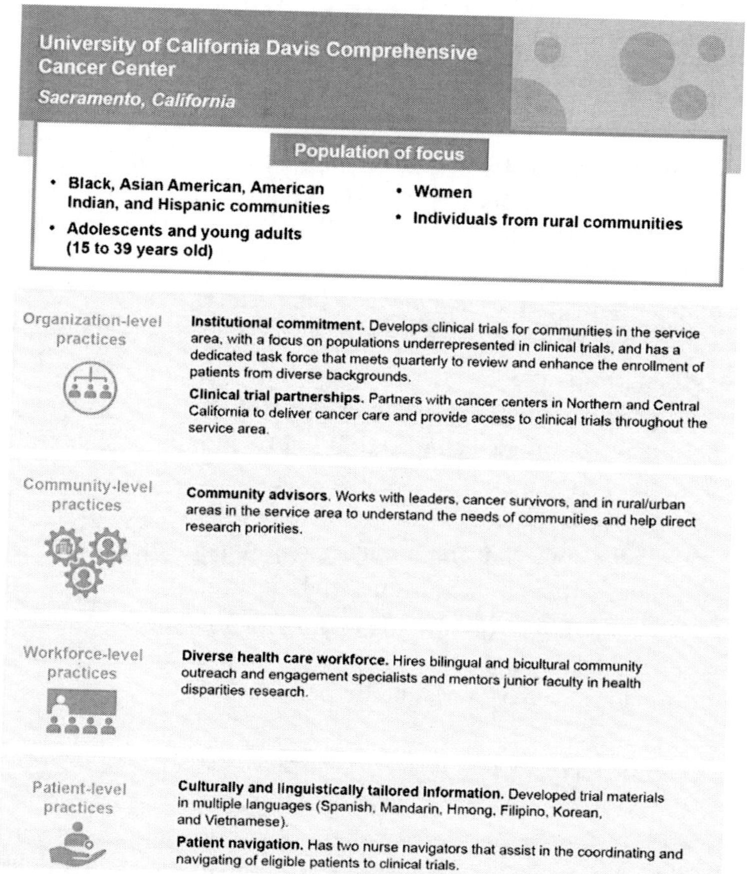

Source: GAO analysis of cancer quiestionnarie responces and other public information. | GAO-23-105245.

Figure 14. Selected University of California at Davis Practices to Facilitate Diverse Patient Representation in Clinical Trials.

From 2011 through 2018, the Partnership enrolled 862 patients in clinical trials of which approximately 76 percent (653 patients) were Black patients.

Case Example: Projects Informed by Service Area Demographics

The University of California Davis Comprehensive Cancer Center has developed programs to identify and address cancer disparities and increase clinical trial enrollment among Hispanic and Asian communities within its service area, including the following:

- The Latinos United for Cancer Health Advancement project, which is focused on reducing cancer disparities by identifying community needs and increasing participation in early detection screenings and clinical trials, conducted a population assessment to better understand cancer within Hispanic communities and conducted outreach in the community by participating in local health fairs, church and other community events. According to Center officials, by forming partnerships with local community organizations, the center was able to build trust with patients and better ensure they completed the population assessment which, in turn, increased the Center's ability to identify disparities and develop interventions to address needs.
- The Asian-American Network for Cancer Awareness, Research and Training initiative—which is focused on reducing cancer disparities through community education, workforce and training, and research— developed clinical trial information in Mandarin, Hmong, Filipino, Korean, and Vietnamese to increase access and knowledge of clinical trials and the use of procedures to reduce cancer disparities and related comorbid conditions among Asian Americans. According to Center officials, having materials in a patient's native language helps to increase trust and education among individuals with limited English proficiency and a better understanding of clinical trial information increases trial participation.

Case Example: Partnerships to Help Address Cancer Disparities Through Clinical Trials

The University of New Mexico Cancer Research and Treatment Center partners with the New Mexico Cancer Research Alliance—a statewide collaboration of clinical trial sites—to address cancer disparities through increased cancer clinical trial awareness, access, and participation among diverse communities across New Mexico. To support and monitor the performance of trials conducted at the Center and at partner sites, the Center established a centralized Clinical Research Office. Additionally, the Center implemented a Community Oncology Work Group that includes representatives from partner sites and meets monthly to review trial options to ensure trials opened are aligned with the needs of diverse communities.

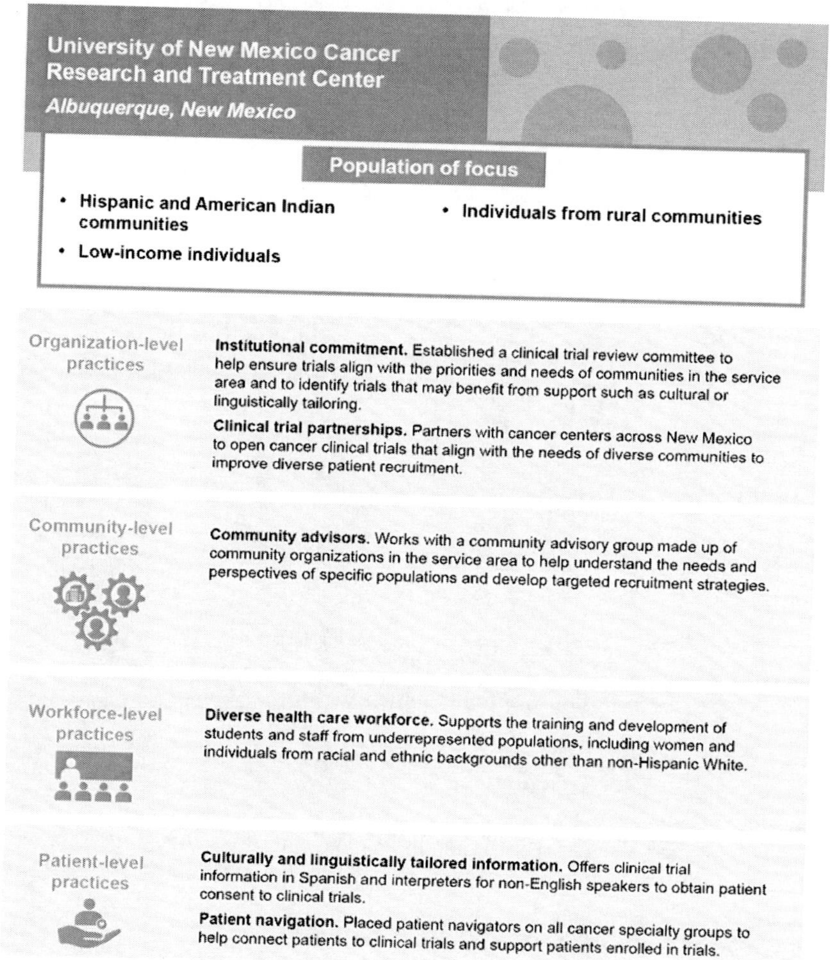

Source: GAO analysis of cancer quiestionnarie responces and other public information. | GAO-23-105245.

Figure 15. Selected University of New Mexico Cancer Research and Treatment Center Practices to Facilitate Diverse Patient Representation in Clinical Trials.

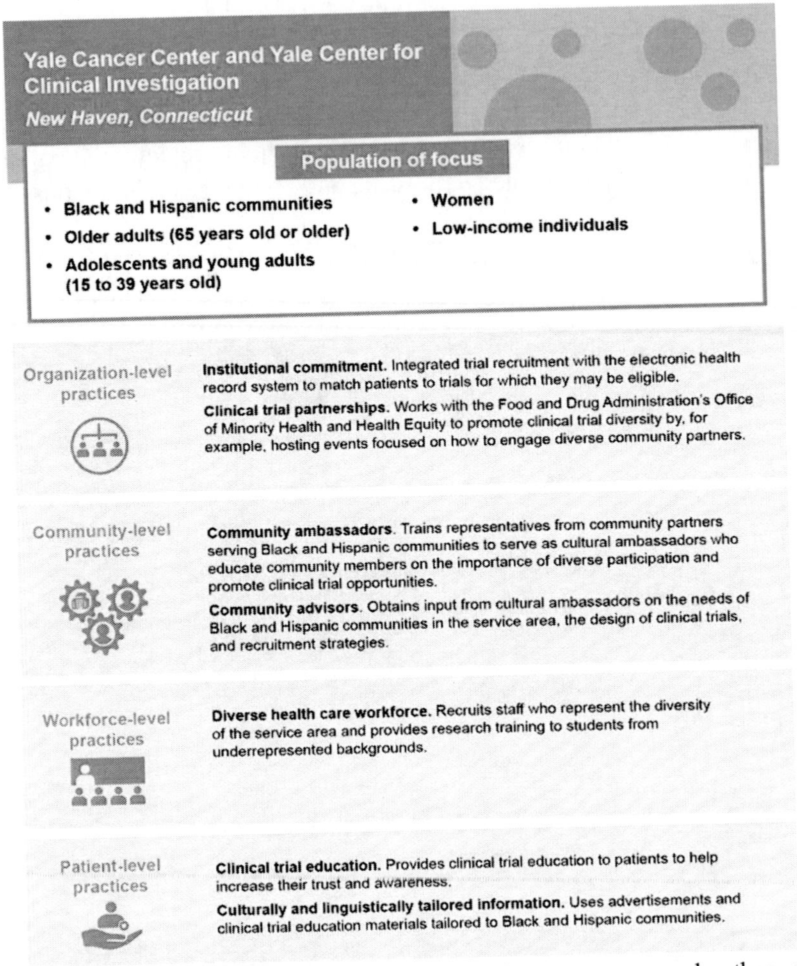

Source: GAO analysis of cancer quiestionnarie responces and other public information. | GAO-23-105245.

Figure 16. Selected Yale Cancer Center and Yale Center for Clinical Investigation Practices to Facilitate Diverse Patient Representation in Clinical Trials.

Case example: Cultural Ambassador Program

Established in 2010, the Yale Center for Clinical Investigation Cultural Ambassador Program is a partnership with the Connecticut African Methodist Episcopal Zion Churches and Junta, organization that serves Hispanic communities in New Haven. Ambassadors are selected by community partners and assist in the development of protocols and recruitment plans for clinical trials and translate information into Spanish. Additionally, ambassadors:

- Promote and increase participation in clinical trials. For example, cultural ambassadors and Yale staff discuss health care issues and how to access clinical trials on two local television shows.
- Support workforce diversity initiatives. For example, Yale staff and cultural ambassadors co-developed a new internship program for high school and undergraduate students to expose and prepare individuals from diverse backgrounds for careers in clinical research.

Center officials reported that, between 2016 and 2021, approximately 61 percent of patients enrolled in trials that involved cultural ambassadors were from racial and ethnic groups other than non-Hispanic White.

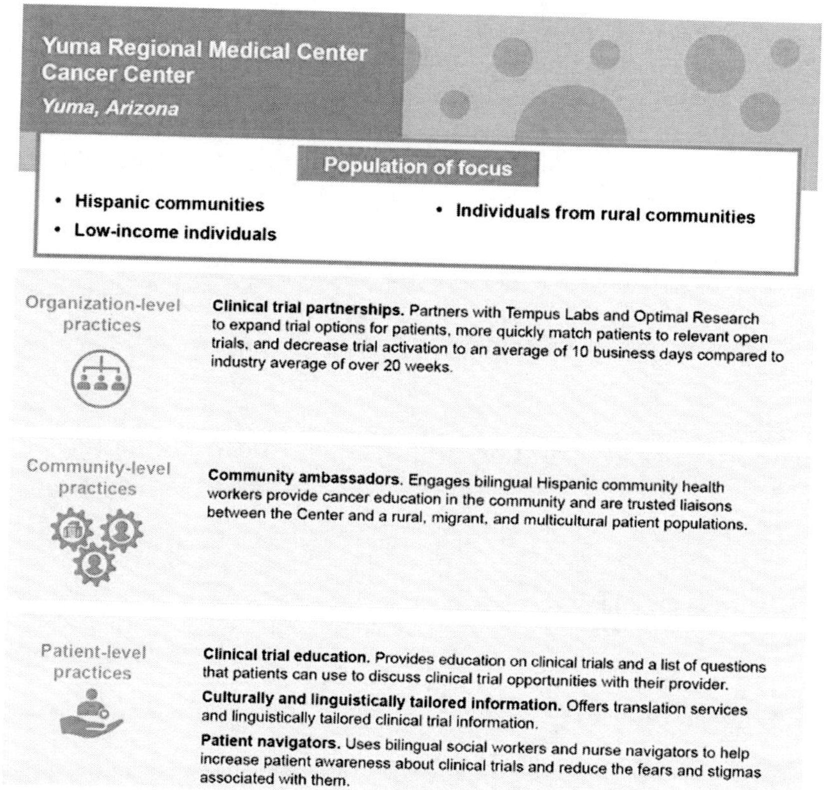

Source: GAO analysis of cancer quiestionnarie responces and other public information. | GAO-23-105245.

Figure 17. Selected Yuma Regional Medical Center Cancer Center Practices to Facilitate Diverse Patient Representation in Clinical Trials.

Case Example: Engaging Hispanic Patients in Cancer Clinical Trials

Yuma Regional Medical Center Cancer Center is located in southwest Arizona and serves a majority Hispanic population. To help ensure Hispanic patients are represented in cancer clinical trials, the Center has taken the following steps:

- Engaged bilingual clinical research staff, social workers, and nurse navigators into patient care and clinical trial outreach to increase awareness of clinical trials and reduce the fears and stigmas associated with them.
- Provided culturally and linguistically tailored clinical trial education for both patients and their caregivers to help increase their understanding of trials.
- Provided patient consent forms are available in multiple languages and formats at the beginning of clinical trial enrollment.
- Employed certified translators so that family members do not have to serve a patient's sole translator and to help enable shared decision-making between patients and their health care providers.

Center officials reported that 39.2 percent of patients enrolled in cancer clinical trials are Hispanic, compared to an average of 3 percent to 6 percent across cancer therapeutic trials more broadly.

Appendix IV: GAO Contact and Staff Acknowledgments

GAO Contacts

John E. Dicken at (202) 512-7114 or DickenJ@gao.gov.

Staff Acknowledgments

In addition to the contacts named above, Jill Center (Assistant Director); Carolyn Feis Korman (Analyst-in-Charge), Derry Henrick and Timothy Kinoshita made key contributions to this report. Also contributing were Ashley Dixon, Keith Haddock, Ruby Samim, Laurie Pachter, Vikki Porter; Emily Wilson Schwark, Cathleen Hamann Whitmore, and Nicole Willis.

GAO's Mission

The Government Accountability Office, the audit, evaluation, and investigative arm of Congress, exists to support Congress in meeting its constitutional responsibilities and to help improve the performance and accountability of the federal government for the American people. GAO examines the use of public funds; evaluates federal programs and policies; and provides analyses, recommendations, and other assistance to help Congress make informed oversight, policy, and funding decisions. GAO's commitment to good government is reflected in its core values of accountability, integrity, and reliability.

Connect with GAO

Connect with GAO on Facebook, Flickr, Twitter, and YouTube. Subscribe to our RSS Feeds or Email Updates. Listen to our Podcasts. Visit GAO on the web at https://www.gao.gov.

To Report Fraud, Waste, and Abuse in Federal Programs

Contact FraudNet:

Website: https://www.gao.gov/about/what-gao-does/fraudnet Automated answering system: (800) 424-5454 or (202) 512-7700

Congressional Relations

A. Nicole Clowers, Managing Director, ClowersA@gao.gov, (202) 512-4400, U.S. Government Accountability Office, 441 G Street NW, Room 7125, Washington, DC 20548.

Public Affairs

Chuck Young, Managing Director, youngc1@gao.gov, (202) 512-4800.

U.S. Government Accountability Office, 441 G Street NW, Room 7149 Washington, DC 20548.

Strategic Planning and External Liaison

Stephen J. Sanford, Managing Director, spel@gao.gov, (202) 512-4707.
U.S. Government Accountability Office, 441 G Street NW, Room 7814, Washington, DC 20548.

Chapter 8

Study on the Incidence of Cancer Diagnosis and Mortality Among Military Aviators and Aviation Support Personnel*

Department of Defense

1. Executive Summary

Introduction

This report is in response to section 750 of the William M. (Mac) Thornberry National Defense Authorization Act (NDAA) for Fiscal Year 2021 (FY) (Public Law 116–283), "Study on the Incidence of Cancer Diagnosis and Mortality among Military Aviators and Aviation Support Personnel." The Act mandated a study on the incidence of cancer diagnosis and mortality among military fixed wing aviators (aircrew) and aviation support personnel (ground crew). This report presents the findings from the Phase 1-a study, which observed that military aircrew and ground crew were overall more likely to be diagnosed with cancer, but less likely to die from cancer compared to the U.S. population. A Phase 1-b study has been initiated which includes additional data from the Department of Veterans Affairs Central Cancer Registry (VACCR) as well as data from 46 State cancer registries. The findings from the Phase 1-a study and implications for the Phase 2 study are provided below.

* This is an edited, reformatted and augmented version of Department of Defense Publication, dated January 2023.

In: Understanding Cancer
Editor: Angela C. Ray
ISBN: 979-8-89530-769-4

Background

- Section 750 of the NDAA for FY 2021 establishes a two-phase study framework.
- Phase 1 requires an epidemiologic study to determine if there is a higher incidence of cancers occurring for military aircrew and ground crew as compared to the U.S. population using the Surveillance, Epidemiology, and End Results (SEER) program database, after adjusting for age, sex, and race.
- If the Phase 1 determination is that there is an increased rate of cancers among military aircrew or ground crew, a second phase is required.
- Most epidemiologic studies have not found a significant difference in rates of cancer diagnosis or death among military aircrew compared to peers in the U.S. population or the U.S. military.
- Few studies have been published on cancer diagnosis or death rates among military ground crew.
- All types of malignant cancer diagnoses were included in this study. However, the following 12 cancers were analyzed separately: colon and rectum, pancreas, melanoma, prostate, testis, urinary bladder, kidney and renal pelvis, brain and other nervous system, thyroid, non-Hodgkin lymphoma, female breast, and lung and bronchus.

Results

- There were 156,050 aircrew and 737,891 ground crew included and followed in the study between 1992 and 2017.
- Military members in both occupational groups were predominantly male and non- Hispanic White, Active Component, and of enlisted rank at entry into the study. Aircrew had a higher proportion of officers compared to ground crew.
- Reserve and National Guard members are more likely to have missing data for cancer diagnoses, therefore, Reserve and National Guard members were excluded from the cancer incidence analysis. Appendix C presents the cancer incidence analysis that includes data from Reserve and National Guard members. In contrast, Reserve and

National Guard member data remained in the cancer mortality analysis.

- The median age at the end of follow-up for the cancer incidence analysis was 41 years for aircrew and 26 years for ground crew. The median age at the end of follow-up for the cancer mortality analysis was 48 years for aircrew and 41 years for ground crew.
- The majority of the aircrew group consisted of members from the Air Force (70.6 percent) and Navy (21.1 percent). The ground crew group also consisted mostly of members from the Air Force (47.8 percent) and Navy (38.3 percent).
- About one-half (50.7 percent, n = 79,124) of the aircrew group and less than one-third (31.4 percent, n = 231,763) of the ground crew group consisted of individuals who joined military service prior to 1990. A small proportion of aircrew (3.5 percent, n = 5,429) and ground crew (3.0 percent, n = 21,852) joined military service in the 1960s or earlier.
- Compared to a demographically similar U.S. population in SEER, aircrew had an 87 percent higher rate of melanoma, 39 percent higher rate of thyroid cancer, 16 percent higher rate of prostate cancer, and a 24 percent higher rate of cancer for all sites combined.
- Ground crew members had higher rates of cancers of brain and nervous system (by 19 percent), thyroid (by 15 percent), melanoma (by 9 percent), kidney and renal pelvis (by 9 percent), and of all sites combined (by 3 percent) compared to the demographically similar U.S. population in SEER.
- Aircrew had a 56 percent lower mortality rate for all cancer sites when compared to the demographically similar U.S. population, and ground crew had a 35 percent lower mortality rate.

Discussion

- The finding that aircrew members had higher rates of melanoma and prostate cancer is similar to previous studies. However, the finding of a higher rate of thyroid cancer has not been previously described.
- This is the first time that cancer risk of all sites has been evaluated in a large population of military ground crew personnel. Comparison

with previous studies is limited due to the scarce amount of prior research in cancer risk among ground crew populations.

- The finding of lower mortality rates in aircrew and ground crew compared to the U.S. population is similar to the findings of other similar studies.
- It is important to note that the military study population was relatively young compared to the U.S. population. Results may have differed if additional older former Service members had been included in the study, since cancer risk and mortality rates increase with age.
- A 2021 Air Force fighter pilot study included all Air Force personnel with active duty service dating back to 1970. Not all of these Air Force members were included in the present study since standardized personnel data back to 1970 were not available for all service branches.
- Results should be interpreted in the context of the study's limitations, with the primary limitation being that this study likely underreported the number of military cancer cases since data from the Department of Veterans Affairs (VA) and civilian cancer registries were not included.
- Although not specifically required by section 750 of the NDAA for FY 2021, an augmentation to the phase 1 study is needed prior to initiating a phase 2 study. This "Phase 1-b study" will supplement the cancer incidence analysis using data from the Virtual Pooled Registry Cancer Linkage System (VPR-CLS) and the VACCR. Including these two data sources will result in better ascertainment of cancer cases for veterans, Reserve and National Guard members, and others without access to TRICARE coverage. A Phase 2 study is required to investigate and identify the specific occupational and environmental risk factors associated with the increased risk of the cancers identified in the Phase 1 study.

2. Purpose of Report – Section 750 of the NDAA for FY 2021 Tasking

Section 750 of the NDAA for FY 2021 contained the following tasking:

SEC. 750. STUDY ON THE INCIDENCE OF CANCER DIAGNOSIS AND MORTALITY AMONG MILITARY AVIATORS AND AVIATION SUPPORT PERSONNEL.

(a) STUDY.—

(1) IN GENERAL. — The Secretary of Defense, in conjunction with the Directors of the National Institutes of Health and the National Cancer Institute, shall conduct a study on cancer among covered individuals in two phases as provided in this subsection.

(2) PHASE 1.—

(A) IN GENERAL. — Under the initial phase of the study conducted under paragraph (1), the Secretary of Defense shall determine if there is a higher incidence of cancers occurring for covered individuals as compared to similar age groups in the general population through the use of the database of the Surveillance, Epidemiology, and End Results (SEER) program of the National Cancer Institute.

(B) REPORT. — Not later than one year after the date of the enactment of this Act, the Secretary shall submit to the appropriate committees of Congress a report on the findings of the initial phase of the study under subparagraph (A).

(3) PHASE 2. —

(A) IN GENERAL. — If, pursuant to the initial phase of the study under paragraph (2), the Secretary concludes that there is an increased rate of cancers among covered individuals, the Secretary shall conduct a second phase of the study under which the Secretary shall do the following:

(i) Identify the carcinogenic toxins1 or hazardous materials associated with military flight operations from shipboard or land bases or facilities, such as fuels, fumes, and other liquids.

(ii) Identify the operating environments, including frequencies or electromagnetic fields, where exposure to ionizing radiation (associated with high altitude flight) and nonionizing radiation (associated with airborne, ground, and shipboard radars) occurred in which covered individuals could have received increased radiation amounts.

(iii) Identify, for each covered individual, duty stations, dates of service, aircraft flown, and additional duties (including Landing Safety Officer, Catapult and Arresting Gear Officer, Air Liaison Officer, Tactical Air Control Party, or personnel associated with aircraft maintenance, supply, logistics, fuels, or transportation) that could have increased the risk of cancer for such covered individual.

(iv) Determine locations where a covered individual served or additional duties of a covered individual that are associated with higher incidences of cancers.

(v) Identify potential exposures due to service in the Armed Forces that are not related to aviation, such as exposure to burn pits or toxins[1] in contaminated water, embedded in the soil, or inside bases or housing.

(vi) Determine the appropriate age to begin screening covered individuals for cancer based on race, gender, flying hours, period of service as aviation support personnel, Armed Force, type of aircraft, and mission.

(B)DATA. — The Secretary shall format all data included in the study conducted under this paragraph in accordance with the Surveillance, Epidemiology, and End Results program of the National Cancer Institute, including by disaggregating such data by race, gender, and age.

(C) REPORT. — Not later than one year after the submittal of the report under paragraph (2)(B), if the Secretary conducts the second phase of the study under this paragraph, the Secretary shall submit to the appropriate committees of Congress a report on the findings of the study conducted under this paragraph.

(4) USE OF DATA FROM PREVIOUS STUDIES. — In conducting the study under this subsection, the Secretary of Defense shall incorporate data from previous studies conducted by the Air Force, the Navy, or the Marine Corps that are relevant to the study under this subsection, including data from the comprehensive study conducted by the Air Force identifying each covered individual and documenting the cancers, dates of diagnoses, and mortality of each covered individual.

(b) DEFINITIONS. — In this section:

(1) The term ‘‘appropriate committees of Congress’’ means—

(A) the Committee on Armed Services and the Committee on Veterans' Affairs of the Senate; and

(B) the Committee on Armed Services and the Committee on Veterans' Affairs of the House of Representatives.

(2) The term ‘‘Armed Forces’’—

(A) has the meaning given the term ‘‘armed forces’’ in section 101 of title 10, United States Code; and

(B) includes the reserve components named in section 10101 of such title.

(3) The term ‘‘covered individual’’—

---

1 The term "toxin" is written in the FY2021 NDAA Sec. 750, but the presumed meaning is "toxicant."

(A) means an aviator or aviation support personnel who— (i) served in the Armed Forces on or after February 28, 1961; and

(ii) receives benefits under chapter 55 of title 10, United States Code; and

(B) includes any aircrew member of fixed-wing aircraft and personnel supporting generation of the aircraft, including pilots, navigators, weapons systems operators, aircraft system operators, personnel associated with aircraft maintenance, supply, logistics, fuels, or transportation, and any other crew member who regularly flies in an aircraft or is required to complete the mission of the aircraft.

2.1. Department of Defense Response

A task force was assembled to conduct the requested study under the oversight of the Defense Health Agency (DHA) and Office of the Deputy Assistant Secretary of Defense for Health Readiness Policy and Oversight within the Office of the Assistant Secretary of Defense for Health Affairs. Representatives from the Service branches, the Armed Forces Health Surveillance Division (AFHSD), National Cancer Institute (NCI), North American Association of Central Cancer Registries (NAACCR), Uniformed Services University of the Health Sciences, and the Murtha Cancer Center participated. The task force established smaller working groups to identify appropriate military data sources, to identify the military study population, and to conduct the analyses for the report.

2.2. Study Strategy

To answer the questions posed by the section 750 of the NDAA for FY 2021 requirement, a two- phase study strategy was mandated:

Phase 1: Conduct an epidemiologic study to determine if there is a higher incidence of cancers occurring among fixed-wing aviators, hereafter referred to as "aircrew", and aviation support personnel, hereafter referred to as "ground crew," compared to the U.S. population using the SEER database after adjusting for age, sex, and race. This phase was led by AFHSD and assisted by NCI, NAACCR, and Service representatives.

Phase 2: Phase 2 is required to be conducted if, under Phase 1, there is determined to be an increased rate of cancers or cancer mortality among military aircrew and ground crew. Phase 2 would consist of identifying the carcinogenic toxicants or hazardous materials associated with military flight operations; identifying operating environments that could be associated with increased amounts of ionizing and nonionizing radiation; identifying specific duties, dates of service, and types of aircraft flown that could have increased the risk for cancer; identifying duty locations associated with higher incidence of cancers; identifying potential exposures due to military service that are not related to aviation; and determining the appropriate age to begin screening military aircrew and ground crew for cancers.

3. Background

3.1. Epidemiology of Cancer among Aircrew and Ground Crew

Most epidemiologic studies prior to 2020 have not found a significant difference in rates of cancer or death due to cancer among aircrew compared to peers in the U.S. population or in the U.S. military [1-5]. However, there have been some studies indicating an increased likelihood of select cancers including brain, female breast, prostate, testicular, and melanoma skin cancers [6- 16]. Of these, melanoma has been the most consistently found to be higher in incidence among aircrew compared to the general population. A meta-analysis conducted in 2019 indicated that airline pilots and cabin crew had about twice the risk of melanoma compared to the general population, with pilots also being more likely to die from melanoma [10].

The U.S. Air Force School of Aerospace Medicine completed a retrospective cohort study in 2021 comparing cancer incidence and mortality among Air Force fighter aviators who served on active duty between 1970 and 2004 with the U.S. population [17]. In that study, fighter aviators were less likely to be diagnosed with cancer of the colon and rectum, testis, urinary bladder, kidney and renal pelvis, and thyroid and less likely to die from colon and rectum cancer. In contrast, male fighter aviators were both more likely to be diagnosed with and die from melanoma skin cancer, prostate cancer, and non-Hodgkin lymphoma.

Few studies have been published to evaluate rates of cancer or death due to cancer among ground crew personnel. However, the few studies available have generally not indicated any increased risk. A 2019 meta-analysis looked at the association between occupational exposure to radar radiation and all types of cancer among workers, which included military members in airports and on airplanes, and found no significant increase in overall relative risk or mortality of cancer [18]. In addition, a cohort study of over 14,000 aircraft maintenance workers at Hill Air Force Base in Utah between 1952 and 1990 did not find a significant increase in cancer incidence or mortality compared to the Utah general population [19]. Another cohort study that followed over 40,000 Navy veterans of the Korean War with radar exposure found no evidence of increased brain or testicular cancer deaths when followed for over 40 years [20].

4. Report of Phase 1-A Study of Cancer Incidence and Mortality

4.1. Background

The objective of the Phase 1-a study is to determine whether there is a higher incidence of cancer diagnosis or mortality among aircrew or ground crew, compared to similar age, sex, and race groups in the U.S. population using the NCI's SEER database. The study protocol for Phase 1-a was approved and determined to be "Not Research" by the DHA Office of Human Research Protections on July 27, 2021.

4.2. Methods

4.2.1. Data Sources

Personnel records were obtained from the Defense Manpower Data Center demographic records maintained in the Defense Medical Surveillance System (DMSS) at the AFHSD. DMSS includes occupational records of all members of the Navy, Air Force, and Marine Corps serving in the active, Reserve, and National Guard Components of the U.S. Armed Forces dating back to 1990 and for Army active, Reserve, and National Guard Components dating back to 1985.

SEER is the authoritative source for cancer incidence and mortality statistics for the U.S., and individuals in this database served as the reference group in the study. Mortality data for the U.S. population originated from the National Center for Health Statistics and are released by SEER. The SEER incidence data date back to 1975 and are currently complete through the end of 2018. However, records did not become standardized using Hispanic and non-Hispanic race/ethnicity categories until 1992.

Cancer cases for the military cohort were identified using the Department of Defense's (DoD) cancer registry system Oncolog, formerly known as the Automated Central Tumor Registry, which is overseen by the DHA's Joint Pathology Center. Oncolog includes cancer data reported by military medical treatment facilities on all DoD beneficiaries, including active-duty military personnel, retired military personnel, and Reserve and National Guard personnel diagnosed while on active duty. These data date back to the mid-1980s but are not considered complete until 1990. At the time of the report, Oncolog data were complete through the end of 2017.

Cancer cases for the military cohort were also identified from the DMSS, which includes inpatient and outpatient administrative (i.e., billing) data for cancer diagnoses that occurred in direct care (i.e., in a military treatment facility) and outsourced care (when reimbursed by TRICARE).

Deaths due to cancer for the military cohort were identified from National Death Index (NDI) Plus data. NDI Plus is the central repository for deaths occurring in the U.S. since January 1979. At the time of request, death records were available through the end of 2018. NDI Plus was accessed through the Joint Department of Veterans Affairs and DoD Suicide Data Repository.

4.2.2. Study Population

Current and former aircrew and ground crew personnel were identified using duty military occupation specialty (DMOS) codes in DMSS. Individuals were included in the study population if: 1) they had an occupation code listed in DMSS, and 2) they were in military service or had an inpatient or outpatient medical encounter at a military treatment facility between 1992 and 2017. Examples of individuals who would be included or not included in the study population are provided in Figure 1. The blue bar in the figure indicates the amount of follow-up time for that individual during the surveillance period.

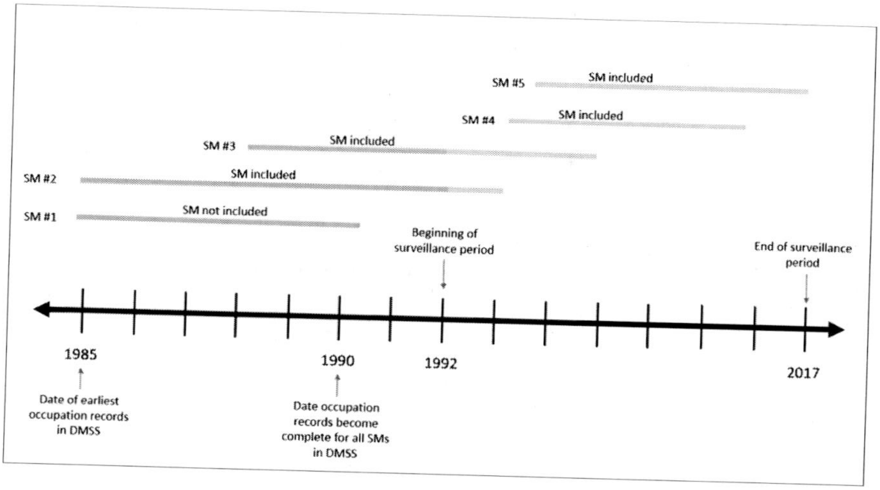

Figure 1. Examples of Service members (SMs) included and not included in the military study population.

The DMOS codes used to identify aircrew and ground crew were selected by Service representatives and subject matter experts. DMOS records specific to remotely piloted aircraft, helicopters or tiltrotor aircraft were excluded. Because not all Navy DMOS codes distinguished between fixed-wing and helicopter aircrew occupations, Navy DMOS records that occurred in tandem with a Unit Identification Code pertaining to helicopter squadrons were also excluded.

Individuals who spent at least 3 years of military service in an aircrew occupation (not including training time) were classified as aircrew. The remaining individuals were then classified according to the occupation category for which they spent the greatest amount of time in during military service, from the time that personnel data became available in DMSS through the end of the study period. For example, if an individual spent 2 years in aircrew occupations, 1.5 years in ground crew occupations, and 1 year in other occupations, they were classified as aircrew. This categorization was determined by subject matter experts to be the best method for identifying enough aircrew members within reason, after inspection of the data and in the absence of information on flight hours. The methodology also draws from the "usual occupation" approach used by the National Institute for Occupational Safety and Health for occupational epidemiology, which was used in a previous study of malignancy in U.S. Air Force fighter pilots [4].

4.2.3. Outcomes

January 1, 1992 was selected as the start date of follow-up for the study and is the date that the SEER database began using standardized race/ethnicity categories, which was necessary for the analysis. December 31, 2017 was selected as the study period end date because it is the period through which Oncolog tumor registry data were considered complete.

All types of malignant cancer diagnoses were included in this study. However, the following 12 cancers were also analyzed separately: colon and rectum, pancreas, melanoma, prostate, testis, urinary bladder, kidney and renal pelvis, brain and other nervous system, thyroid, non-Hodgkin lymphoma, female breast, and lung and bronchus. These cancers were selected based on concern from veteran advocacy groups and prior cancer studies that demonstrated increased incidence in military populations. DoD cancer cases from Oncolog were categorized according to SEER site recoding instructions available at: https://seer.cancer.gov/siterecode/icdo3_dwhoheme/index.html.

Oncolog data primarily only includes cases identified in military treatment facilities. DMSS data were included so that cancer cases diagnosed in outsourced care reimbursed by TRICARE would also be identified. Inpatient data are available in DMSS back to 1990 and outpatient data are available back to 1996. Administrative data case-finding algorithms were used to identify incident cancer cases in the DMSS data [21]. The list of qualifying International Classifications of Diseases, 9th and 10th edition (ICD-9 and ICD-10) diagnoses by cancer type can be found in Appendix B. In a previous study, a standardized chart review was conducted to validate the AFHSD DMSS case-finding algorithms and found the algorithms work well for prostate, testis, and thyroid cancers, and for melanoma [23]. However, diagnoses for the gall bladder, small intestine, larynx, miscellaneous, "other" male or female genital organs, and "other" digestive system were excluded from the analysis because the AFHSD algorithm is not good at identifying those types of cancers (positive predictive value ≤ 50 percent), and those cases would be likely not to be true cancer cases [23]. In addition, DMSS-identified cancers of brain and nervous system, lung and bronchus, bones and joints, and liver cancers were excluded if they occurred after another cancer case of a different site, because these cases were likely to be metastases and not true incident cancers [22].

NDI Plus mortality data were obtained from the Defense Suicide Prevention Office. The underlying cause of death was assigned to a cancer category based on ICD codes consistent with SEER cause of death recode available at https://seer.cancer.gov/codrecode/.

4.2.4. Analysis

For the cancer incidence analysis, two separate analyses were performed: 1) Oncolog and DMSS cancer cases combined, with Reserve and National Guard members excluded from the study population; and 2) Oncolog and DMSS cancer cases combined, with Reserve and National Guard members included. The results of the first analysis are emphasized in this report because Reserve/National Guard members are more likely to seek care outside of the military health system and therefore less likely to be picked up as a case. As a result, including Reserve and National Guard members could bias the results of the study towards seeing no risk for cancer or seeing reduced risk of cancer when that might not be true. Oncolog and DMSS cancer cases were combined because cases in Oncolog may be underreported, particularly for individuals after they leave military service.

For all analyses, cancer cases, cancer deaths, and person-time in the military study population was assigned to unique combinations (called "stratum") for race/ethnicity (Non-Hispanic White, Non-Hispanic Black, Hispanic, and Other), sex (male, female), and age group category (5-year intervals). Person-time for the cancer incidence analysis was estimated by calculating the time from the earliest date of military service through the latest date of military service or last medical encounter reimbursed by TRICARE. If cancer was diagnosed after the last medical encounter or date in service, then the follow-up period was extended to the date of the cancer diagnosis.

Person-time was counted from the beginning of the study period on January 1, 1992, to the end of the study period on December 31, 2017.

NCI investigators calculated the observed number of U.S. population cases and population sizes for each stratum using SEER. SEER uses mid-year population estimates as a proxy for the person-time at risk in the calendar year, and multiple tumors may be counted as cases in the numerator. The number of expected cases is the cases that would be expected to occur in the military cohort had they experienced the same age, sex, and race stratum-specific risks of the U.S. population. The number of expected cases was calculated by AFHSD using the SEER stratum-specific rates, and this expected number of cases was compared to the number of observed cases for the military cohort. This analysis comparing observed to expected number of cases was performed separately for aircrew and ground crew.

Similar calculations were performed for the mortality analysis, which measured the occurrence of death due to malignant cancer of all sites as well as the 12 site-specific cancers. The person- time at risk for death started on January 1, 1992, or at entry into the study population (i.e., first date of military service). It ended at the end of the study period on December 31, 2017, or at the time of death due to any cause. This person-time differed from the incidence analysis because NDI Plus covers all deaths in the United States, and therefore it was expected that deaths occurring in individuals in the military study population could be identified at any point during the surveillance period. All Active, Reserve, and National Guard military Components were included in the mortality analysis since they would all be expected to be included in the NDI Plus data.

Standardized incidence ratios (SIRs) were calculated as the number of observed over the number of expected incident cancer cases (see Appendix D). These ratios were calculated separately for malignant cancer of all sites, for each of the 12 specific cancers, and separately for aircrew and ground crew. Standardized mortality ratios (SMRs) were also calculated for deaths due to malignant cancer of all sites, for each of the 12 listed cancers, and separately for each of the military sub-cohorts. Finally, 95 percent confidence intervals and p-values were generated using a Poisson distribution. All statistical analyses were performed using SAS® software (Version 9.4, SAS Inst, Inc., Cary, NC).

4.3. Results

4.3.1. Introduction

This section describes the military study population, and then presents the results of the two cancer incidence analyses. The results of the first incidence analysis, in which Reserve and National Guard members were excluded, is presented first. The results of the second incidence analysis, in which Reserve and National Guard members were included, is presented second. Finally, the results from the cancer mortality analysis are presented, which includes both active and Reserve/National Guard Component members.

4.3.2. Description of Military Study Population

There were 156,050 aircrew and 737,891 ground crew included in the military cohort, which included both Active and Reserve/National Guard Component members (Table 1). Follow-up time varied depending on the analysis being conducted (see person years in Tables 2-5 and Appendix C tables). Service members in both aircrew and ground crew were predominantly male and non-Hispanic White, Active Component, aged 29 or less at entry into the study, and of enlisted rank at entry. However, aircrew had a higher proportion of officers compared to ground crew, with 49.8 percent enlisted and 48.9 percent officer. The majority of the aircrew group consisted of members from the Air Force (70.6 percent), followed by the Navy (21.1 percent).

The ground crew group also consisted mostly of members from the Air Force (47.8 percent) and Navy (38.3 percent). About one-half (50.7 percent, n = 79,124) of the aircrew group and less than one-third (31.4 percent, n = 231,763) of the ground crew group consisted of individuals who joined military service prior to 1990. A small proportion of aircrew (3.5 percent, n = 5,429) and ground crew (3.0 percent, n=21,852) joined military service in the 1960s or earlier.

4.3.3. Age at Follow-up, Diagnosis, and Death

For the cancer incidence analysis (Reserve/National Guard members excluded), the median age at the end of follow-up for malignant cancer of all sites was 41 years for aircrew and 26 years for ground crew. For the cancer mortality analysis, the median age at the end of follow-up for malignant cancer of all sites was 48 years for aircrew and 41 years for ground crew (Reserve/National Guard members included).

The median age at diagnosis for malignant cancer of all sites (Reserve/National Guard members excluded) was 54 years in aircrew and 53 years in ground crew. In contrast, the median age at diagnosis for malignant cancer of all sites was 67 years in the SEER reference population. The median age at death for malignant cancer of all sites was 57 in aircrew and 56 years in ground crew (Reserve/National Guard members included). In the SEER reference population, the median age at death for malignant cancer of all sites was 72 years.

Table 1. Demographics of the military study cohort

	Aircrew		Ground crew	
	N	%	N	%
Total study population	156,050	100	737,891	100
Age (years)[a]				
29 or less	109,235	70.0	602,835	81.7
30-49	45,778	29.3	128,465	17.4
50+	1,037	0.67	6,591	0.9
Sex				
Male	145,385	93.2	664,782	90.1
Female	10,665	6.8	73,109	9.9
Race/ethnicity				

Table 1. (Continued)

	Aircrew		Ground crew	
	N	%	N	%
Non-Hispanic White	134,839	86.4	527,747	71.5
Non-Hispanic Black	6,666	4.3	90,279	12.2
Hispanic	7,953	5.1	69,865	9.5
Non-Hispanic Other	6,592	4.2	50,000	6.8
Service[a]				
Army	4,067	2.6	41,501	5.6
Navy	32,866	21.1	282,701	38.3
Air Force	110,225	70.6	352,307	47.8
Marine Corps	8,892	5.7	61,382	8.3
Component[a]				
Active	128,682	82.5	598,334	81.1
Reserve	14,885	9.5	76,673	10.4
National Guard	12,483	8.0	62,884	8.5
Rank[a]				
Enlisted	77,781	49.8	719,068	97.5
Officer	76,269	48.9	9,738	1.3
Missing/ unknown	2,000	1.3	9,085	1.2
Year at entry into military service				
1940-1949	6	0.0	25	0.0
1950-1959	371	0.2	2,530	0.3
1960-1969	5,052	3.2	19,297	2.6
1970-1979	26,499	17.0	72,729	9.9
1980-1989	47,196	30.2	137,182	18.6
1990-1999	33,059	21.2	193,135	26.2
2000-2009	33,037	21.2	184,979	25.1
2010-2017	10,467	6.7	122,606	16.6
Missing/unknown[b]	363	0.2	5,408	0.7

[a] Age, service branch, Component, and rank were measured at the beginning of follow-up.

[b] Year at entry was defined as missing/unknown for individuals aged <17 years or > 45 years at the date of entry into military service, as these were assumed to be data entry errors.

4.3.4. Cancer Incidence: Military Compared to U.S. Population

Oncolog and DMSS-Defined Cancer Cases: Reserve/National Guard Members Excluded

There was a total of 4,639,667 malignant cancer cases observed in SEER during the study period. In the military cohort, there were 6,381 malignant cancer cases among aircrew and 12,246 among ground crew.

After adjusting for age, sex, and race/ethnicity, aircrew members had statistically higher incidence of cancers of all sites (by 24 percent), melanoma (by 87 percent), thyroid (by 39 percent), and prostate (by 16 percent), compared to individuals in the U.S. population (Table 2). Incidence of cancers of the colon and rectum, urinary bladder, kidney and renal pelvis, and lung and bronchus were statistically lower compared to individuals in the U.S. population by 44 percent, 35 percent, 17 percent, and 71 percent, respectively. There was not a statistically significant difference between aircrew members and members of the U.S. population for cancers of the pancreas, testis, brain and nervous system, non-Hodgkin lymphoma, and female breast.

Table 2. Observed and expected cancer cases, aircrew compared to U.S. population, 1992-2017

Cancer site	Person-years	Observed cases	Expected cases	SIR	95% LL	95% UL	p- value
All sites	1,664,080	6,381	5,155	1.24	1.21	1.27	<.0001
Colon and rectum	1,710,570	282	502	0.56	0.50	0.63	<.0001
Pancreas	1,712,278	103	117	0.88	0.72	1.07	0.2079
Melanoma	1,704,826	802	429	1.87	1.74	2.00	<.0001
Prostate	1,625,276	1,542	1,331	1.16	1.10	1.22	<.0001
Testis	1,632,177	196	178	1.10	0.95	1.27	0.1896
Urinary bladder	1,711,338	175	270	0.65	0.56	0.75	<.0001
Kidney and renal pelvis	1,711,281	191	229	0.83	0.72	0.96	0.0107
Brain and nervous system	1,711,872	122	122	1.00	0.83	1.19	1.0000
Thyroid	1,710,520	180	129	1.39	1.20	1.61	<.0001
Non-Hodgkin lymphoma	1,710,287	298	301	0.99	0.88	1.11	0.8752
Female breast	76,832	59	51	1.16	0.88	1.49	0.2949
Lung and bronchus	1,711,977	164	563	0.29	0.25	0.34	<.0001

Ground crew members had statistically higher incidence of cancer of all sites (by 3 percent), brain and nervous system (by 19 percent), thyroid (by 15 percent), melanoma (by 9 percent), and kidney and renal pelvis (by 9 percent), compared to individuals in the U.S. population (Table 3). Ground crew members had statistically lower incidence of cancers of the colon and rectum (by 25 percent), prostate (by 5 percent), urinary bladder (by 10 percent), and lung and bronchus (by 24 percent). There was no statistically significant difference for cancers of the pancreas, testis, female breast, and non-Hodgkin lymphoma.

Table 3. Observed and expected cancer cases, ground crew compared to U.S. population, 1992-2017

Cancer site	Person-years	Observed cases	Expected cases	SIR	95% LL	95% UL	p- value
All sites	5,023,723	12,246	11,909	1.03	1.01	1.05	0.0022
Colon and rectum	5,100,002	842	1,125	0.75	0.70	0.80	<.0001
Pancreas	5,104,970	240	257	0.93	0.82	1.06	0.3033
Melanoma	5,097,646	937	859	1.09	1.02	1.16	0.0093
Prostate	4,689,565	2,694	2,845	0.95	0.91	0.98	0.0045
Testis	4,700,826	473	467	1.01	0.92	1.11	0.7811
Urinary bladder	5,102,468	463	516	0.90	0.82	0.98	0.0195
Kidney and renal pelvis	5,102,170	559	513	1.09	1.00	1.18	0.0455
Brain and nervous system	5,103,657	340	287	1.19	1.06	1.32	0.0024
Thyroid	5,102,234	369	321	1.15	1.04	1.27	0.0094
Non-Hodgkin lymphoma	5,100,679	667	691	0.97	0.89	1.04	0.3743
Female breast	397,139	239	223	1.07	0.94	1.22	0.3012
Lung and bronchus	5,103,317	800	1,216	0.66	0.61	0.71	<.0001

Oncolog and DMSS-Defined Cancer Cases: Reserve/National Guard Members Included

When Reserve and National Guard members were included, there were 8,491 malignant cancer cases among aircrew and 17,656 among ground crew. After adjusting for age, sex, and race/ethnicity, aircrew members had statistically higher incidence of melanoma (by 63 percent), thyroid cancer (by 19 percent), and cancer of all sites (by 8 percent), compared to individuals in the U.S. population (Appendix Table C1). Incidence of cancers of the colon and rectum, pancreas, testis, urinary bladder, kidney and renal pelvis, brain and nervous system, non- Hodgkin lymphoma, and lung and bronchus were statistically lower compared to individuals in the U.S. population. There was not a statistically significant difference between aircrew members and members of the U.S. population for cancers of the prostate and female breast.

Among ground crew members, incidence of all cancers was statistically lower for ground crew members compared to members of the U.S. population (Appendix Table C2). However, for cancers of the thyroid and brain and nervous system, this difference was not statistically significant.

4.3.5. Cancer Mortality: Military Compared to U.S. Population

During the study period, there were 1,240 deaths due to any malignant cancer among aircrew personnel, 5,784 among ground crew, and 14,471,873 in the U.S. population. After adjusting for age, sex, and race/ethnicity, aircrew members had statistically lower mortality rates due to malignant cancer of all sites (56 percent) when compared to individuals in the general U.S. population (Table 4). Of the 12 cancers that were evaluated separately, aircrew had statistically lower mortality rates due to cancers of the colon and rectum (by 60 percent), pancreas (by 33 percent), prostate (by 34 percent), testis (by 75 percent), urinary bladder (by 52 percent), kidney and renal pelvis (by 40 percent), brain and nervous system (by 24 percent), non-Hodgkin lymphoma (by 58 percent), female breast (by 54 percent), and lung and bronchus (by 74 percent). There was not a statistically significant difference between aircrew and the U.S. population in the mortality rates for melanoma and thyroid cancer.

Table 4. Observed and expected cancer deaths, aircrew compared to U.S. population, 1992-2017

Cancer site	Person- years	Observed deaths	Expected deaths	SMR	95% Lower CI	95% Upper CI	p-value
All sites	3,188,015	1,240	2,832	0.44	0.41	0.46	<.0001
Colon and rectum	3,188,015	107	269	0.40	0.33	0.48	<.0001
Pancreas	3,188,015	112	168	0.67	0.55	0.80	<.0001
Melanoma	3,188,015	76	85	0.90	0.71	1.13	0.3865
Prostate	3,010,539	63	96	0.66	0.50	0.84	0.0004
Testis	3,010,539	3	12	0.25	0.05	0.74	0.0050
Urinary bladder	3,188,015	26	54	0.48	0.32	0.71	<.0001
Kidney and renal pelvis	3,188,015	53	88	0.60	0.45	0.78	<.0001
Brain and nervous system	3,188,015	103	136	0.76	0.62	0.92	0.0038
Thyroid	3,188,015	8	7	1.16	0.50	2.29	0.7681
Non-Hodgkin lymphoma	3,188,015	49	117	0.42	0.31	0.56	<.0001
Female breast	177,476	8	18	0.46	0.20	0.90	0.0182
Lung and bronchus	3,188,015	224	849	0.26	0.23	0.30	<.0001

Similarly, ground crew personnel had a lower mortality rate (by 35 percent) due to malignant cancer of all sites compared to individuals in the general U.S. population (Table 5). Of the 12 cancers that were evaluated separately, ground crew personnel had lower mortality rates due to cancers of the colon and rectum (by 37 percent), pancreas (by 16 percent), prostate (by 43 percent), urinary bladder (by 25 percent), kidney and renal pelvis (by 21 percent), non-Hodgkin lymphoma (by 34 percent), and lung and bronchus (by 46 percent). There was not a statistically significant difference observed between ground crew personnel and the U.S. population in the mortality rates for melanoma, testicular cancer, brain and nervous system cancer, thyroid, and female breast cancer.

Table 5. Observed and expected cancer deaths, ground crew compared to U.S. population, 1992-2017

Cancer site	Person-years	Observed deaths	Expected deaths	SMR	95% Lower CI	95% Upper CI	p- value
All sites	13,274,928	5,784	8,927	0.65	0.63	0.66	<.0001
Colon and rectum	13,274,928	535	852	0.63	0.58	0.68	<.0001
Pancreas	13,274,928	426	510	0.84	0.76	0.92	0.0002
Melanoma	13,274,928	215	241	0.89	0.78	1.02	0.1020
Prostate	12,149,032	190	335	0.57	0.49	0.65	<.0001
Testis	12,149,032	38	46	0.83	0.59	1.14	0.2902
Urinary bladder	13,274,928	120	159	0.75	0.63	0.90	0.0015
Kidney and renal pelvis	13,274,928	208	264	0.79	0.69	0.90	0.0004
Brain and nervous system	13,274,928	390	419	0.93	0.84	1.03	0.1683
Thyroid	13,274,928	15	21	0.71	0.40	1.18	0.2197
Non-Hodgkin lymphoma	13,274,928	250	378	0.66	0.58	0.75	<.0001
Female breast	1,125,896	89	97	0.92	0.74	1.13	0.4602
Lung and bronchus	13,274,928	1,377	2,551	0.54	0.51	0.57	<.0001

5. Discussion

5.1. Summary

This study found that compared to the U.S. population after adjusting for age, sex, and race, aircrew had an 87 percent higher rate of melanoma, 39 percent higher rate of thyroid cancer, 16 percent higher rate of prostate cancer, and a 24 percent higher rate of cancer for all sites. Ground crew members had higher incidence of cancers of brain and nervous system (by 19 percent), thyroid (by 15 percent), melanoma (by 9 percent), kidney and renal pelvis (by 9 percent), and of all sites (by 3 percent). However, aircrew and ground crew both had lower or similar cancer mortality rates for all cancer types when compared to the U.S. population. This concludes the Phase 1-a epidemiologic study required by section 750 of the NDAA for FY 2021 and triggers the Phase 2 study to identify risk factors for cancer diagnosis. Prior to initiation of a Phase 2 study, a Phase 1-b study is being conducted which will include additional data from the VACCR as well as data from 46 state cancer registries.

5.1.1. Cancer Incidence

The finding of increased melanoma cancer rates in aircrew is in line with previous studies that have demonstrated higher incidence of melanoma among aircrew compared to non-aircrew populations [7-8, 10, 15, 24]. However, incidence of melanoma was also elevated in ground crew members (by 9 percent). This suggests that air and ground crew could share risk factors associated with increased risk for or detection of malignant melanoma.

The incidence of thyroid cancer was 39 percent higher among aircrew members and 15 percent higher among ground crew compared to the U.S. population. Previous studies have not found significant elevated risk of thyroid cancer incidence or mortality among airline crew relative to the general population [25]. However, a study comparing military thyroid cancer incidence rates to the U.S. population during 1990-2004 found higher military rates among various racial/ethnic groups [26].

Aircrew members were 16 percent more likely to be diagnosed with prostate cancer, which is similar to findings from the 2021 Air Force study which found that male fighter aviators were 19 percent more likely to be diagnosed with prostate cancer compared to the U.S. population [17]. The reasons for this elevated incidence are not well understood. Studies conducted through 2019 have found an average of 41 percent increased risk of prostate cancer in pilots, although this does not include other flight personnel and there is much variation across studies [27].

Ground crew members had higher rates of diagnosis for cancers of the brain and nervous system (by 19 percent), thyroid (by 15 percent), kidney and renal pelvis (by 9 percent), and melanoma (by 9 percent). This is the first time that cancer risk has been evaluated in such a large population of military ground crew, and comparison with previous studies is limited due to the scarce amount of existing information on the topic.

The incidence of cancer of all sites was higher in aircrew (by 24 percent) and slightly higher in ground crew (by 3 percent) compared to the U.S. population. It is currently unclear which type(s) of cancer(s) are driving this association and further analysis is recommended to determine whether this is due to one or multiple cancer types.

5.1.2. Cancer Mortality

This study did not find a higher cancer mortality rate among aircrew or ground crew compared to the U.S. population. In contrast, the mortality rate for malignant cancer of all sites was significantly lower in aircrew (by 56 percent) and ground crew (by 35 percent). A recent study of cause-specific mortality for U.S. veterans of conflicts in Afghanistan and Iraq between 2001 and 2016 found a 44 percent decreased risk for malignant cancer deaths when compared to the U.S. population after adjusting for age, sex, race, and year [28]. This finding of lower mortality rates in military populations compared to the U.S. population is similar to the results of the present study.

A 2021 Air Force study found that fighter aviators had lower rates of death due to colon and rectum cancer but higher rates of death due to melanoma, prostate cancer, and non-Hodgkin lymphoma [17]. One likely explanation for this difference is the age of the study populations. In the fighter pilot study, the average (mean) age at mortality censoring was 64 years and in the current study it was 47 years for aircrew. Thus, it is possible that the present study lacked sufficient follow-up time for progression to mortality in older age groups.

Previous studies have documented the "healthy soldier effect," which is defined as the proposition that U.S. military members are healthier than the general U.S. population by nature of having to meet military fitness standards [29]. Military members must meet initial physical fitness requirements for accession, maintain and pass periodic fitness tests, and generally have better access to medical care during and after military service. In addition, aircrew members may be required to meet even more stringent physical standards to maintain their flight status. Previous studies have estimated that the healthy soldier effect on cancer mortality is 17-19 percent, meaning that Service members may have a 17-19 percent lower risk of cancer mortality compared to the general population simply by nature of being in the military [29]. However, it has also been suggested that this effect erodes over longer years of follow-up time. In an Australian study of Korea and Vietnam War veterans, cancer mortality rates were similar to those of the general population for the first 20 years of follow-up, but rose between 20 and 30 years post follow-up, and fell back to general population levels after 30 years of follow-up [30]. A study of Royal Norwegian Navy servicemen who served during 1950–2004 reported similar patterns of findings [31].

Another potential partial explanation for why military aircrew or ground crew members could be at higher risk for the diagnosis of certain cancers, but not at higher risk for dying from those cancers, is that Service members have routine medical screenings and physical fitness tests while they are in service. As a result, Service members may be more likely to have some types of cancers detected and diagnosed at earlier stages, thus improving their prognosis. In previous studies, patients diagnosed in the military health system in particular have been shown to have better survival and better screening rates for lung and colon cancer [32-34].

5.2. Study Strengths

This is one of the largest and most comprehensive studies of military aircrew and ground crew cancer risks to-date. Enough women were included in the study that risks for female-specific cancers could be evaluated. The study population includes members who served in different military conflicts over time. By using a standardized data source, the DMSS, the study team was able to quickly identify the study population and adjust for basic demographic factors.

5.3. Study Limitations

5.3.1. Data Availability and Quality

The most significant limitations to this study are related to data availability and quality. Section 750 of the NDAA for FY 2021 defined the military study population as aviators or aviation support personnel who served in the Armed

Forces on or after February 28, 1961, and who receive benefits under chapter 55 of title 10, U.S. Code (which includes Active and Reserve/National Guard Component members). The task force was unable to identify an electronic data source containing information on military occupation and dates of service prior to 1990. The 2021 Air Force fighter aviator study included personnel with active-duty service dating back to 1970, identified by the Air Force Personnel Center. However, not all of these Air Force members were included in the present study since standardized personnel data back to 1970 were not available for all Service branches.

There are known gaps in the military cancer case data. The task force was unable to identify a data source containing complete data on cancer diagnoses prior to 1990. Veterans, Reserve and National Guard members, and others without access to TRICARE coverage are likely missing cancer data, which could bias the results of the study towards seeing no risk for cancer or seeing reduced risk of cancer when that might not be true. In addition, outpatient data were not available in DMSS until 1996, which likely resulted in missing cancer cases as well as an underestimation of follow-up time for cancer in the military cohort. There are some data sources that should have been included in this study in order to have complete ascertainment of all cancer cases for the military cohort; however, 12 months was not enough time to gather these data.

Currently, AFHSD is collaborating with the NAACCR to identify cancer cases for the military study population using the Virtual Pooled Registry Cancer Linkage System (VPR-CLS), which includes U.S. population cancer data from 43 registries across the country between the early 1990s and 2019. AFHSD is also seeking data from the VACCR and together these data sources will provide a more complete count of cancer cases for the military study cohort.

Finally, it should be noted that there were unavoidable differences in the ways that cancer incidence was calculated in the military cohort compared to how incidence was calculated in SEER. SEER uses mid-year population estimates as a proxy for the person-time at risk in the calendar year, and multiple tumors may be counted as cases. However, in the military cohort, rates are calculated by following individuals in the study population over time using person- years, and only the first occurrence of each type of cancer is counted. The effect that this might have had on the final study results is unknown.

5.3.2. Exposure Misclassification

For this Phase 1-a study, DMOS codes were used to identify occupational groups, which has several limitations. Ideally, flight hours and the type of aircraft should be taken into consideration, but these data were not available. In addition, a person's occupation while in military service can change over time. Establishing a causal relationship between a person's military occupation and cancer would require that the exposure (i.e., occupation) or accumulation of exposure to a certain threshold (i.e., years spent in a certain occupation) occurs prior to first cancer diagnosis. The "usual occupation" approach does not take this temporality of exposure and cancer into consideration. Different cancers have different latency periods, which is the time that it takes for cancer to develop following the first exposure to a cancer-causing agent. These latency periods should be taken into consideration but were not for this study.

However, the objective of this study was to compare cancer incidence rates in the military population to those in SEER, and latency periods are also not accounted for in the SEER rates.

Finally, DMOS codes are not standardized across branches, which can lead to variability in the types of occupations selected into the aircrew and ground crew groups. The distinction between aircrew and ground crew was not clearly defined for some DMOS codes, and, because data on flight hours were not available, the determination was made by subject matter experts but may have resulted in some occupational misclassification.

5.3.3. Uncontrolled Confounding Factors

There are multiple risk factors associated with cancer that could not be addressed in the Phase 1- a study. Due to the features of cancer registry and medical claims data, data are not available on family history of cancer, smoking, alcohol use, physical activity, overweight/obesity status, recreational environmental exposures, diet, and other lifestyle factors, which may confound the comparison of cancer incidence and mortality between the military study population and the U.S. population. The "healthy soldier" effect may also confound the results of this study. Since military members tend to be healthier than the general population by nature of being in military service, this may obscure any increased risk of cancer or cancer mortality due to occupational exposures.

5.4. Conclusion

The findings of this study suggest that aircrew and ground crew who served in the military relatively recently have higher incidence of cancer compared to individuals in the U.S. population. This finding cannot be generalized to members who served prior to 1990 because it does not include all members who served prior to this date. It also does not imply that military service in aircrew or ground crew occupations causes cancer, because there are multiple potential confounding factors that could not be controlled for in this analysis. The SIRs and SMRs presented in this report should only be used to compare aircrew to the U.S. population and to compare ground crew to the U.S. population. They should not be used to compare cancer risk and mortality rates between aircrew and ground crew since the methods used do not allow for this comparison. Findings further indicate that military aircrew and ground crew have lower risk of death due to cancer compared to the U.S. population. However, it is important to note that study results may have differed had additional older former Service members been included.

The results should be interpreted in the context of the study's limitations, with the primary limitation being that this study likely underreported the number of military cancer cases since data from VA and civilian cancer registries were not included.

5.5. Way Forward

A supplementary Phase 1-b study is being conducted prior to initiating a Phase 2 study in order to augment the cancer incidence analysis using data from the VPR-CLS and the VACCR. This will allow the inclusion of data from veterans, Reserve, and National Guard members. The VPR-CLS is a new system designed to connect state cancer registries across the U.S. It has not yet been used for large military or VA cancer studies, and this study will be the first. An initial query through VPR-CLS identified thousands of cancer cases available for data extraction in 46 state cancer registries. Section 750 of the NDAA for FY 2021 states that Phase 2 shall be conducted if, under Phase 1, there is determined to be an increased rate of cancers among military aircrew and ground crew. Given the findings of higher incidence for some cancers among aircrew and ground crew in the Phase 1 study, the Phase 2 study is required. Phase 2 will consist of identifying the carcinogenic toxicants or hazardous materials associated with military flight operations; identifying operating environments that could be associated with increased amounts of ionizing and nonionizing radiation; identifying specific duties, dates of service, and types of aircraft flown that could have increased the risk for cancer; identifying duty locations associated with higher incidence of cancers; identifying potential exposures due to military service that are not related to aviation; and determining the appropriate age to begin screening military aircrew and ground crew for cancers.

References

[1] Langner I., Blettner M., Gundestrup M., et al. Cosmic radiation and cancer mortality among airline pilots: results from a European cohort study (ESCAPE). *Radiat. Environ. Biophys.* 2004;42(4):247-256. doi:10.1007/ s00411-003-0214-7.

[2] Hammer G.P., Blettner M., Langner I., Zeeb H. Cosmic radiation and mortality from cancer among male German airline pilots: extended cohort follow-up. *Eur. J. Epidemiol.* 2012;27(6):419-429. doi:10.1007/ s10654-012-9698-2.

[3] Sigurdson A. J., Ron E. Cosmic radiation exposure and cancer risk among flight crew. *Cancer Invest.* 2004;22(5):743-61. doi: 10.1081/cnv-200032767. PMID: 15581056.

[4] Robbins A. S., Pathak S. R., Webber B. J., Erich R. A., Escobar J. D., Simon A. A., et al. (2020) Malignancy in U.S. Air Force fighter pilots and other officers, 1986–2017: A retrospective cohort study. *PLoS ONE* 15(9): e0239437. https://doi.org/10.1371/journal.pone.0239437.

[5] Rogers D., Boyd D. D., Fox E. E., et al. Prostate cancer incidence in U.S. Air Force aviators compared with non-aviators. *Aviat Space Environ. Med.* 2011;82(11):1067-1070. doi:10.3357/asem.3090.2011.

[6] Sigurdson A. J., Ron E. Cosmic radiation exposure and cancer risk among flight crew. *Cancer Invest.* 2004;22(5):743-61. doi: 10.1081/cnv-20003 2767 . PMID: 15581056.

[7] Hammar N., Linnersjö A., Alfredsson L., Dammström B. G., Johansson M., Eliasch H. Cancer incidence in airline and military pilots in Sweden 1961-1996. *Aviat. Space Environ. Med.* 2002 Jan;73(1):2-7. PMID: 11817615.

[8] Haldorsen T., Reitan J. B., Tveten U. Cancer incidence among Norwegian airline pilots. *Scand. J. Work Environ. Health.* 2000 Apr;26(2):106-11. doi: 10.5271/sjweh.519. PMID: 10817375.

[9] Buja A., Lange J. H., Perissinotto E., et al. Cancer incidence among male military and civil pilots and flight attendants: an analysis on published data. *Toxicol. Ind. Health.* 2005;21(10):273-282. doi:10.1191/ 0748233705th 238oa.

[10] Miura K., Olsen C. M., Rea S., Marsden J., Green A. C. Do airline pilots and cabin crew have raised risks of melanoma and other skin cancers? Systematic review and meta-analysis. *Br. J. Dermatol.* 2019 Jul;181(1):55-64. doi: 10.1111/bjd.17586. Epub 2019 Mar 18. PMID: 30585313.

[11] Pukkala E., Aspholm R., Auvinen A., et al. Cancer incidence among 10,211 airline pilots: a Nordic study. *Aviat. Space Environ. Med.* 2003;74(7):699-706.

[12] Grayson J. K., Lyons T. J. Cancer incidence in United States Air Force aircrew, 1975-89. *Aviat. Space Environ. Med.* 1996 Feb;67(2):101-4. PMID: 883 4932.

[13] Grayson J. K., Lyons T. J. Brain cancer, flying, and socioeconomic status: a nested case- control study of USAF aircrew. *Aviat. Space Environ. Med.* 1996 Dec;67(12):1152-4. PMID: 8968480.

[14] Ballard T., Lagorio S., De Angelis G., Verdecchia A. Cancer incidence and mortality among flight personnel: a meta-analysis. *Aviation, Space, and Environmental Medicine.* 2000 Mar;71(3):216-224.

[15] Sanlorenzo M., Wehner M. R., Linos E., et al. The risk of melanoma in airline pilots and cabin crew: a meta-analysis. *JAMA Dermatol.* 2015;151(1):51-58. doi:10.1001/jamadermatol.2014.1077.

[16] McNeely E., Mordukhovich I., Staffa S., et al. Cancer prevalence among flight attendants compared to the general population. *Environ. Health.* 2018 Jun 26;17(1):49. doi: 10.1186/s12940-018-0396-8. PMID: 29940975; PMCID: PMC6019786.

[17] Webber B. J., Tacke C. D., Wolff G. G., et al. Cancer Incidence and Mortality Among Fighter Aviators in the United States Air Force. *J. Occup. Environ. Med.* 2022;64(1):71-78. doi:10.1097/JOM.0000000000002353.

[18] Safari Variani A., Saboori S., Shahsavari S., Yari S., Zaroushani V. Effect of Occupational Exposure to Radar Radiation on Cancer Risk: A Systematic Review and Meta-Analysis. *Asian Pac. J. Cancer Prev.* 2019;20(11):3211-3219. Published 2019 Nov 1. doi:10.31557/ APJCP.2019.20.11.3211.

[19] Blair A., Hartge P., Stewart P. A., et al. Mortality and cancer incidence of aircraft maintenance workers exposed to trichloroethylene and other organic solvents and chemicals: extended follow up. *Occupational and Environmental Medicine* 1998;55:161- 171.

[20] Groves F. D., Page W. F., Gridlcy G, et al. Cancer in Korean war navy technicians: mortality survey after 40 years. *Am. J. Epidemiol.* 2002;155(9):810-818. doi:10.1093/aje/155.9.810.

[21] Armed Forces Health Surveillance Division. Surveillance Case Definitions. https://health.mil/Military-Health-Topics/Combat-Support/ Armed-Forces-Health-Surveillance-Division/Epidemiology-and-Analysis/Surveillance-Case-Definitions.

[22] NAACCR Death Clearance Working Group. Death Clearance Manual: Minimum Requirements and Best Practices for Conducting Death Clearance. Springfield, IL: North American Association of Central Cancer Registries, January 2010. https://www.naaccr.org/wp- content/uploads/ 2020/04/DC_Manual_Appendix_I_updated_Final_04162020-1.pdf.

[23] Webber BJ, Rogers AE, Pathak SR, Robbins AS. Positive predictive value of an algorithm used for cancer surveillance in the U.S. Armed Forces. MSMR. 2019 Dec;26(12):18-22. PMID: 31860325.

[24] Brundage J. F., Williams V. F., Stahlman S., McNellis M. G. Incidence rates of malignant melanoma in relation to years of military service, overall and in selected

military occupational groups, Active Component, U.S. Armed Forces, 2001-2015. MSMR. 2017;24(2):8-14.
[25] Liu, G. S., Cook, A., Richardson, M. et al. Thyroid cancer risk in airline cockpit and cabin crew: a meta-analysis. *Cancers Head Neck* 3, 7 (2018). https://doi.org/10.1186/s41199- 018-0034-8.
[26] Enewold L. R., Zhou J., Devesa S. S., et al. Thyroid cancer incidence among active duty U.S. military personnel, 1990-2004. *Cancer Epidemiol. Biomarkers Prev.* 2011;20(11):2369- 2376. doi:10.1158/1055-9965.EPI-11-0596.
[27] Krstev S., Knutsson A. Occupational Risk Factors for Prostate Cancer: A Meta-analysis. *J. Cancer Prev.* 2019;24(2):91-111. doi:10.15430/ JCP.2019. 24.2.91.
[28] Bullman T., Schneiderman A. Cause-Specific mortality risks through 2016, among U.S. veterans of the Southwest Asia Theater. *Journal of Military and Veterans' Health.* 2021;29(3):52-56.
[29] McLaughlin R., Nielsen L., Waller M. An evaluation of the effect of military service on mortality: quantifying the healthy soldier effect [published correction appears in *Ann. Epidemiol. 2015 Feb;25(2):143]. Ann. Epidemiol.* 2008;18(12):928-936. doi:10.1016/j.annepidem. 2008. 09.002.
[30] Waller M., McGuire A. C. Changes over time in the "healthy soldier effect". *Popul. Health Metr*. 2011;9:7. Published 2011 Mar 14. doi:10.1186/1478-7954-9-7.
[31] Strand L. A., Martinsen J. I., Fadum E. A., et al. Temporal trends in the healthy soldier effect in a cohort of Royal Norwegian Navy servicemen followed for 67 years. *Occupational and Environmental Medicine* 2020; 77:775-781.
[32] Bytnar J. A., Shriver C. D., Zhu K. Incidence rates of digestive cancers among U.S. military servicemen: Comparison with the rates in the general U.S. population. *PLoS One.* 2021;16(9):e0257087. Published 2021 Sep 3. doi:10.1371/journal.pone.0257087.
[33] Lin J., Kamamia C., Brown D., et al. Survival among Lung Cancer Patients in the U.S. Military Health System: A Comparison with the SEER Population. *Cancer Epidemiol. Biomarkers Prev.* 2018;27(6):673-679. doi:10.1158/1055-9965.EPI-17-0822.
[34] Weygandt, J., Robling, K., Whitaker, L. A., McPherson, K., Hartwell, M., & Greiner, B. (2021). Cancer Screening Among Current and Former U.S. Military Personnel Compared to Civilians: A Cross-Sectional Analysis of the Behavioral Risk Factor Surveillance System. *Military medicine,* usab439. Advance online publication. https://doi.org/ 10.1093/milmed/ usab439.

Appendix A: Acronyms

AFHSD	Armed Forces Health Surveillance Division
CI	Confidence Interval
DHA	Defense Health Agency
DMOS	duty military occupational specialty

DMSS	Defense Medical Surveillance System
DoD	Department of Defense
FY	Fiscal Year
ICD	International Classification of Diseases
NAACCR	North American Association of Central Cancer Registries
NCI	National Cancer Institute
NDI	National Death Index
NDAA	National Defense Authorization Act
SEER	Surveillance, Epidemiology, and End Results
SIR	standardized incidence ratio
SMR	standardized mortality ratio
USAF	U.S. Air Force
VA	Department of Veterans Affairs
VACCR	Veterans Affairs Central Cancer Registry
VPR-CLS	Virtual Pooled Registry Cancer Linkage System

Appendix B: ICD-9 and ICD-10 Diagnosis Codes Used to Identify DMSS Cancer Cases

	ICD-9-CM	*ICD-10-CM*
Lip	140	C00
Tongue	141	C01, C02
Salivary gland	142	C07, C08
Floor of mouth	144	C04
Gum and other mouth	143, 145	C03, C05, C06
Nasopharynx	147	C11
Tonsil	1460-1462	C09
Oropharynx	1463-1469	C10
Hypopharynx	148	C12, C13
Other Oral Cavity and Pharynx	149	C14
Esophagus	150	C15
Stomach	151	C16
Small intestine	152	C17
Colon and rectum	153, 1540-1541, 1590	C18-C20, C260
Anus, Anal Canal and Anorectum	1542-1543, 1548	C21
Liver	1550, 1552	C220, C222- C229
Intrahepatic Bile Duct	1551	C221
Gallbladder	1560	C23
Other Biliary	1561-1562, 1568-1569	C24

	ICD-9-CM	*ICD-10-CM*
Pancreas	157	C25
Retroperitoneum	1580	C480
Peritoneum, Omentum and Mesentery	1588-1589	C451, C481, C482
Other Digestive Organs	1598-1599	C268-C269, C488
Nose, Nasal Cavity and Middle Ear	160	C30, C31
Larynx	161	C32
Lung and Bronchus	1622-1625, 1628-1629	C34
Pleura	163	C384, C450
Trachea, Mediastinum and Other Respiratory Organs	1620, 1642-1643, 1648-1649, 165	C33, C381-C383, C388, C39
Bones and Joints	170	C40, C41
Soft Tissue including Heart	1641, 171	C47, C49, C380, C452
Melanoma (of the Skin)	172	C43
Non-Melanoma (Skin)	173	C44
Breast	174, 175	C50
Cervix Uteri	180	C53
Corpus Uteri	182	C54
Uterus, NOS	179	C55
Ovary	1830	C56
Vagina	1840	C52
Vulva	1841-1844	C51
Other Female Genital Organs	181, 1832-1835, 1838-1839, 1848-1849	C57, C58
Prostate	185	C61
Testis	1860, 1869	C620, C621, C629
Penis	1871-1874	C60
Other Male Genital Organs	1875-1879	C63
Urinary bladder	188	C67
Kidney and renal pelvis	1890-1891	C64-C65
Ureter	1892	C66
Other Urinary Organs	1893-1894, 1898-1899	C68
Eye and Orbit	190	C69
Brain and other nervous system	191, 192	C70, C71, C72
Thyroid	193	C73
Other Endocrine including Thymus	1640, 194	C37, C74, C75
Hodgkin Lymphoma	201	C81
Non-Hodgkin lymphoma	200, 2020-2022, 2027-2029	C82–C86, C96Z, C969
Myeloma	2030, 2386	C900, C902, C903
Acute Lymphocytic Leukemia	2040	C910
Chronic Lymphocytic Leukemia	2041	C911

Appendix B. (Continued)

	ICD-9-CM	*ICD-10-CM*
Other Lymphocytic Leukemia	2024, 2042, 2048-2049	C912-C914, C916-C919, C91A, C91Z
Acute myeloid	2050, 2070, 2072	C920, C924-C926, C928, C940, C942, C92A
Acute Monocytic Leukemia	2060	C930
Chronic Myeloid Leukemia	2051	C921
Other Myeloid/Monocytic Leukemia	2052-2053, 2058-2059, 2061-2062, 2068-2069	C922-C923, C927, C929, C931-C933, C937, C939, C92Z, C93Z
Other Acute Leukemia	2080	C944, C950
Aleukemic, subleukemic and NOS	2031, 2071, 2078, 2081-2082, 2088-2089	C901, C915, C941, C943, C947, C951, C959, C948
Mesothelioma	N/A	C45
Kaposi Sarcoma	176	C46
Miscellaneous Malignant Cancer	1591, 195-199, 2023, 2025-2026, 2038	C261, C457, C459, C76- C80, C88, C946, C960- C962, C964-C968, C97

Appendix C

Table C1. Observed and expected cancer cases (Oncolog and DMSS data), aircrew compared to U.S. population, 1992-2017. Reserve and National Guard members are included

Cancer site	Person- years	Observed cases	Expected cases	SIR	95% LL	95% UL	p- value
All sites	2,619,013	8,491	7,834	1.08	1.06	1.11	<.0001
Colon and rectum	2,678,236	386	753	0.51	0.46	0.57	<.0001
Pancreas	2,680,464	136	174	0.78	0.65	0.92	0.0031
Melanoma	2,671,020	1,073	656	1.63	1.54	1.74	<.0001
Prostate	2,531,071	2,030	1,950	1.04	1.00	1.09	0.0716
Testis	2,540,401	247	285	0.87	0.76	0.98	0.0251
Urinary bladder	2,679,172	241	406	0.59	0.52	0.67	<.0001
Kidney and renal pelvis	2,679,321	243	342	0.71	0.62	0.81	<.0001

Cancer site	Person- years	Observed cases	Expected cases	SIR	95% LL	95% UL	p- value
Brain and nervous system	2,679,999	159	188	0.85	0.72	0.99	0.0356
Thyroid	2,678,310	242	203	1.19	1.05	1.35	0.0080
Non-Hodgkin lymphoma	2,677,955	391	459	0.85	0.77	0.94	0.0012
Female breast	136,027	90	96	0.94	0.76	1.16	0.6083
Lung and bronchus	2,680,098	223	839	0.27	0.23	0.30	<.0001

Table C2. Observed and expected cancer cases (Oncolog and DMSS data), ground crew compared to U.S. population, 1992-2017. Reserve and National Guard members are included

Cancer site	Person- years	Observed cases	Expected cases	SIR	95% LL	95% UL	p- value
All sites	7,312,190	17,656	20,677	0.85	0.84	0.87	<.0001
Colon and rectum	7,416,703	1,187	1,958	0.61	0.57	0.64	<.0001
Pancreas	7,423,422	352	462	0.76	0.68	0.85	<.0001
Melanoma	7,413,612	1,345	1,437	0.94	0.89	0.99	0.0153
Prostate	6,844,069	4,307	5,342	0.81	0.78	0.83	<.0001
Testis	6,864,627	559	676	0.83	0.76	0.90	<.0001
Urinary bladder	7,419,461	757	1,009	0.75	0.70	0.81	<.0001
Kidney and renal pelvis	7,419,708	784	864	0.91	0.85	0.97	0.0062
Brain and nervous system	7,421,983	415	454	0.91	0.83	1.01	0.0668
Thyroid	7,420,425	448	490	0.91	0.83	1.00	0.0589
Non-Hodgkin lymphoma	7,417,921	918	1,140	0.81	0.75	0.86	<.0001
Female breast	550,761	289	327	0.89	0.79	0.99	0.0373
Lung and bronchus	7,421,054	1,179	2,276	0.52	0.49	0.55	<.0001

Appendix D

Standardized Incidence Ratio (SIR)

The SIR is a ratio of the number of observed cancer cases in the military aircrew and ground crew compared to the number that would be expected to occur in the aircrew and ground crew if they experienced the same cancer rates at the U.S. population. The SIR adjusts for differences in age, sex, and race/ethnicity.

$$SIR = \frac{Observed\ Cancer\ Cases\ (O)}{Expected\ Cancer\ Cases\ (E)}$$

Standardized Mortality Ratio (SMR)

The SMR is a ratio of the number of observed cancer deaths in the military aircrew and ground crew compared to the number that would be expected to occur in the aircrew and ground crew if they experienced the same cancer mortality rates at the U.S. population. The SMR adjusts for differences in age, sex, and race/ethnicity.

$$SMR = \frac{Observed\ Cancer\ Deaths\ (O)}{Expected\ Cancer\ Deaths\ (E)}$$

UNDER SECRETARY OF DEFENSE
4000 DEFENSE PENTAGON
WASHINGTON, D.C. 20301-4000

The Honorable Mike D. Rogers
Chairman
Committee on Armed Services
U.S. House of Representatives
Washington, DC 20515

Dear Mr. Chairman:

The Department's response to section 750 of the William M. (Mac) Thornberry National Defense Authorization Action Act (NOAA) for Fiscal Year (FY) 2021 (Public Law 116-283), "Study on the Incidence of Cancer Diagnosis and Mortality Among Military Aviators and Aviation Support Personnel," is enclosed. Section 750(a)(2)(8) requests a report on the results of Phase I of the study, which determines ifthere is a higher incidence of cancers occurring for these military aviators and aviation support personnel as compared to similar age groups in the general population through the use of the database of the Surveillance, Epidemiology, and End Results program of the National Cancer Institute.

This study found that compared to the U.S. population after adjusting for age, sex, and race, aircrew had an 87 percent higher rate of melanoma, 39 percent higher rate of thyroid cancer, 16 percent higher rate of prostate cancer, and a 24 percent higher rate of cancer for all sites. Ground crew members had higher incidence of cancers of brain and nervous system (by 19 percent), thyroid (by 15 percent), melanoma (by 9 percent), kidney and renal pelvis (by 9 percent), and of all sites (by 3 percent). However, aircrew and ground crew both had lower or similar cancer mortality rates for all cancer types when compared to the U.S. population. This concludes the Phase 1 epidemiologic study and triggers a Phase 2 study to identify risk factors for the cancer diagnoses identified in the Phase 1 study. Elements to be included in the Phase 2 study are outlined in section 750(a)(3)(c) of the NOAA for FY 2021.

There are known gaps in military cancer case data with no Department of Defense data source containing complete data on cancer diagnoses prior to 1990. This has likely resulted in the Phase 1-a study having underreported the number of military cancer cases since data from the Department of Veterans Affairs (VA) and civilian cancer registries were not included. This lack of cancer data on veterans, Reserve, and National Guard members could bias the results of this Phase 1-a study. To address this limitation, prior to initiating the Phase 2 study, a supplementary Phase 1-b study is being conducted including additional data from the VA and 46 State cancer registries. This Phase 1-b study will supplement the cancer incidence analysis using data from the VA Central Cancer Registry and the Virtual Pooled Registry Cancer Linkage System.

Including these two data sources will result in better ascertainment of cancer cases for veterans, Reserve, and National Guard members, and others without access to TRICARE coverage.

Thank you for your continued strong support for the health and well-being of our Service members, veterans, and their families. I am sending similar letters to the appropriate committees of Congress.

Sincerely,

Gilbert R. Cisneros, Jr.

Enclosure:
As stated

cc:
The Honorable Adam Smith Ranking Member

The Honorable Jack Reed
Chairman
Committee on Armed Services
United States Senate
Washington, DC 20510

Dear Mr. Chairman:

The Department's response to section 750 of the William M. (Mac) Thornberry National Defense Authorization Action Act (NDAA) for Fiscal Year (FY) 2021 (Public Law 116-283), "Study on the Incidence of Cancer Diagnosis and Mortality Among Military Aviators and Aviation Support Personnel," is enclosed. Section 750(a)(2)(B) requests a report on the results of Phase 1 of the study, which determines if there is a higher incidence of cancers occurring for these military aviators and aviation support personnel as compared to similar age groups in the general population through the use of the database of the Surveillance, Epidemiology, and End Results program of the National Cancer Institute.

This study found that compared to the U.S. population after adjusting for age, sex, and race, aircrew had an 87 percent higher rate of melanoma, 39 percent higher rate of thyroid cancer, 16 percent higher rate of prostate cancer, and a 24 percent higher rate of cancer for all sites. Ground crew members had higher incidence of cancers of brain and nervous system (by 19 percent), thyroid (by 15 percent), melanoma (by 9 percent), kidney and renal pelvis (by 9 percent), and of all sites (by 3 percent). However, aircrew and ground crew both had lower or similar cancer mortality rates for all cancer types when compared to the U.S. population. This concludes the Phase 1 epidemiologic study and triggers a Phase 2 study to identify risk factors for the cancer diagnoses identified in the Phase 1 study. Elements to be included in the Phase 2 study are outlined in section 750(a)(3)(c) of the NDAA for FY 2021.

There are known gaps in military cancer case data with no Department of Defense data source containing complete data on cancer diagnoses prior to 1990. This has likely resulted in the Phase 1-a study having underreported the number of military cancer cases since data from the Department of Veterans Affairs (VA) and civilian cancer registries were not included. This lack of cancer data on veterans, Reserve, and National Guard members could bias the results of this Phase 1-a study. To address this limitation, prior to initiating the Phase 2 study, a supplementary Phase 1-b study is being conducted including additional data from the VA and 46 State cancer registries. This Phase 1-b study will supplement the cancer incidence analysis using data from the VA Central Cancer Registry and the Virtual Pooled Registry Cancer Linkage System.

Including these two data sources will result in better ascertainment of cancer cases for veterans, Reserve, and National Guard members, and others without access to TRICARE coverage.

Thank you for your continued strong support for the health and well-being of our Service members, veterans, and their families. I am sending similar letters to the appropriate committees of Congress.

Sincerely,

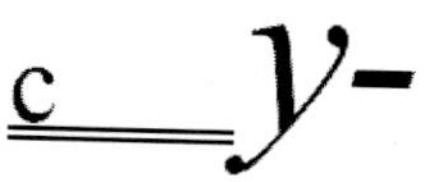

Gilbert R. Cisneros, Jr.

Enclosure:
As stated

cc:
The Honorable Roger F. Wicker, Ranking Member

The Honorable Jon Tester
Chairman
Committee on Veterans' Affairs United States Senate
Washington, DC 20510

Dear Mr. Chairman:

The Department's response to section 750 of the William M. (Mac) Thornberry National Defense Authorization Action Act (NDAA) for Fiscal Year (FY) 2021 (Public Law 116-283), "Study on the Incidence of Cancer Diagnosis and Mortality Among Military Aviators and Aviation Support Personnel," is enclosed. Section 750(a)(2)(B) requests a report on the results of Phase 1 of the study, which determines if there is a higher incidence of cancers occurring for these military aviators and aviation support personnel as compared to similar age groups in the general population through the use of the database of the Surveillance, Epidemiology, and End Results program of the National Cancer Institute.

This study found that compared to the U.S. population after adjusting for age, sex, and race, aircrew had an 87 percent higher rate of melanoma, 39 percent higher rate of thyroid cancer, 16 percent higher rate of prostate cancer, and a 24 percent higher rate of cancer for all sites. Ground crew members had higher incidence of cancers of brain and nervous system (by 19 percent), thyroid (by 15 percent), melanoma (by 9 percent), kidney and renal pelvis (by 9 percent), and of all sites (by 3 percent). However, aircrew and ground crew both had lower or similar cancer mortality rates for all cancer types when compared to the U.S. population. This concludes the Phase 1 epidemiologic study and triggers a Phase 2 study to identify risk factors for the cancer diagnoses identified in the Phase 1 study. Elements to be included in the Phase 2 study are outlined in section 750(a)(3)(c) of the NDAA for FY 2021.

There are known gaps in military cancer case data with no Department of Defense data source containing complete data on cancer diagnoses prior to 1990. This has likely resulted in the Phase 1-a study having underreported the number of military cancer cases since data from the Department of Veterans Affairs (VA) and civilian cancer registries were not included. This lack of cancer data on veterans, Reserve, and National Guard members could bias the results of this Phase 1-a study. To address this limitation, prior to initiating the Phase 2 study, a supplementary Phase 1-b study is being conducted including additional data from the VA and 46 State cancer registries. This Phase 1-b study will supplement the cancer incidence analysis using data from the VA

Central Cancer Registry and the Virtual Pooled Registry Cancer Linkage System.

Including these two data sources will result in better ascertainment of cancer cases for veterans, Reserve, and National Guard members, and others without access to TRICARE coverage.

Thank you for your continued strong support for the health and well-being of our Service members, veterans, and their families. I am sending similar letters to the appropriate committees of Congress.

Sincerely,

Gilbert R. Cisneros, Jr.

Enclosure:
As stated

cc:
The Honorable Jerry Moran, Ranking Member

The Honorable Mike Bost Chairman
Committee on Veterans' Affairs
U.S. House of Representatives
Washington, DC 20515

Dear Mr. Chairman:

The Department's response to section 750 of the William M. (Mac) Thornberry National Defense Authorization Action Act (NDAA) for Fiscal Year (FY) 2021 (Public Law 116-283), "Study on the Incidence of Cancer Diagnosis and Mortality Among Military Aviators and Aviation Support Personnel," is enclosed. Section 750(a)(2)(B) requests a report on the results of Phase 1 of the study, which determines ifthere is a higher incidence of cancers occurring for these military aviators and aviation support personnel as compared to similar age groups in the general population through the use of the database of the Surveillance, Epidemiology, and End Results program of the National Cancer Institute.

This study found that compared to the U.S. population after adjusting for age, sex, and race, aircrew had an 87 percent higher rate of melanoma, 39 percent higher rate of thyroid cancer, 16 percent higher rate of prostate cancer, and a 24 percent higher rate of cancer for all sites. Ground crew members had higher incidence of cancers of brain and nervous system (by 19 percent), thyroid (by 15 percent), melanoma (by 9 percent), kidney and renal pelvis (by 9 percent), and of all sites (by 3 percent). However, aircrew and ground crew both had lower or similar cancer mortality rates for all cancer types when compared to the U.S. population. This concludes the Phase 1 epidemiologic study and triggers a Phase 2 study to identify risk factors for the cancer diagnoses identified in the Phase 1 study. Elements to be included in the Phase 2 study are outlined in section 750(a)(3)(c) of the NDAA for FY 2021.

There are known gaps in military cancer case data with no Department of Defense data source containing complete data on cancer diagnoses prior to 1990. This has likely resulted in the Phase 1-a study having underreported the number of military cancer cases since data from the Department of Veterans Affairs (VA) and civilian cancer registries were not included. This lack of cancer data on veterans, Reserve, and National Guard members could bias the results of this Phase 1-a study. To address this limitation, prior to initiating the Phase 2 study, a supplementary Phase 1-b study is being conducted including additional data from the VA and 46 State cancer registries. This Phase 1-b study will supplement the cancer incidence analysis using data from the VA Central Cancer Registry and the Virtual Pooled Registry Cancer Linkage System.

Including these two data sources will result in better ascertainment of cancer cases for veterans, Reserve, and National Guard members, and others without access to TRICARE coverage.

Thank you for your continued strong support for the health and well-being of our Service members, veterans, and their families. I am sending similar letters to the appropriate committees of Congress.

Sincerely,

Gilbert R. Cisneros, Jr.

Enclosure:
As stated

cc:
The Honorable Mark Takano, Ranking Member

Chapter 9

Women and Lung Cancer Research and Preventive Services Act of 2024*

Committee on Energy and Commerce

The Committee on Energy and Commerce, to whom was referred the bill (H.R. 4534) to require a review of women and lung cancer, and for other purposes, having considered the same, reports favorably thereon with an amendment and recommends that the bill as amended do pass.

The amendment is as follows:

Strike all after the enacting clause and insert the following:

SECTION 1. SHORT TITLE.

This Act may be cited as the "Women and Lung Cancer Research and Preventive Services Act of 2024."

SEC. 2. INTERAGENCY REVIEW TO EVALUATE AND IDENTIFY OPPORTUNITIES FOR THE ACCELERATION OF RESEARCH ON LUNG CANCER IN WOMEN AND UNDERSERVED POPULATIONS, GREATER ACCESS TO PREVENTIVE SERVICES, AND STRATEGIC PUBLIC AWARENESS AND EDUCATION CAMPAIGNS.

(a) IN GENERAL. — The Secretary of Health and Human Services, in consultation with the Secretary of Defense and Secretary of Veterans Affairs, shall conduct an interagency review to evaluate the status of, and identify opportunities related to—

(1) research on lung cancer in women;

---

* This is an edited, reformatted and augmented version of Report of Mrs. Rodgers of Washington, from the Committee on Energy and Commerce Committed to the Committee of the Whole House on the State of the Union and ordered to be printed, Publication No. 118–622, dated July 30, 2024.

In: Understanding Cancer
Editor: Angela C. Ray
ISBN: 979-8-89530-769-4

(2) research on lung cancer in underserved populations that meet the eligibility criteria for lung cancer screening as recommended by the United States Preventive Services Task Force;

(3) access to lung cancer preventive services; and

(4) strategic public awareness and education campaigns on lung cancer.

(b) CONTENT.—The review and recommendations under subsection (a) shall include—

(1) a review and comprehensive report on the outcomes of previous research, the status of existing research activities, and knowledge gaps related to lung cancer in women and underserved populations in all agencies of the Federal Government;

(2) opportunities for collaborative, interagency, multidisciplinary, and innovative research, that would—

(A) encourage innovative approaches to eliminate knowledge gaps in research on lung cancer in women;

(B) evaluate environmental and genomic factors that may be related to the etiology of lung cancer in women; and

(C) foster advances in imaging technology and techniques to improve risk assessment, diagnosis, treatment, and the simultaneous utilization of other preventive services and activities;

(3) opportunities regarding the development of a national lung cancer screening strategy to expand access to such screenings, particularly among women and underserved populations; and

(4) opportunities regarding the development of a national public education and awareness campaign on—

(A) lung cancer in women and underserved populations; and

(B) the importance of early detection of lung cancer.

(c) REPORT. — Not later than two years after the date of the enactment of this Act, the Secretary of Health and Human Services shall submit to Congress a report on the review conducted under subsection (a).

Purpose and Summary

H.R. 4534 requires The Department of Health and Human Services (HHS) to conduct an interagency review on the status of, and identify research related to, women and underserved populations with lung cancer. The review would include assessments of current research and access to prevention services, the availability of research opportunities regarding prevention, detection, and treatment, and recommendations for national public education and screening strategies.

Background and Need for Legislation

Lung cancer is the third most common cancer in the United States.[1] Worldwide, over 600,000 women die of lung cancer each year.[2] About 10 to 20 percent of lung cancers, or 20,000 to 40,000 lung cancers each year, happen in people who never smoked or smoked fewer than 100 cigarettes in their lifetime.[3] A better under standing of additional risk factors beyond smoking cigarettes is needed for more effective screening, diagnosis, and treatment.

H.R. 4534 would review and assess current research on lung cancer in women and certain underserved populations, as well as evaluate current relevant opportunities related to education and access to prevention, detection, and treatment services.

Committee Action

On February 14, 2024, the Subcommittee on Health held a hearing on H.R. 4534. The title of the hearing was "Legislative Proposals to Support Patients and Caregivers." The Subcommittee received testimony from:

- Andy Shih, PhD, Chief Science Officer, Autism Speaks;
- Corey Feist, JD, MBA, Co-Founder and CEO, Dr. Lorna Breen Heroes' Foundation;
- Joanne Pike, DrPH, President and CEO, Alzheimer's Association;
- Gordon Tomaselli, MD, Former President, American Heart Association; Marilyn and Stanley M. Katz Dean, Emeritus and

---

[1] "Lung Cancer Statistics," U.S. Centers for Disease Control and Prevention, June 13, 2024, https://www.cdc.gov/lung-cancer/statistics/?CDC_AAref_Val=https://www.cdc.gov/cancer/lung/statistics/index.htm.

[2] "Women and Lung Cancer," Lung Cancer Research Foundation, https://www.lungcancerresearchfoundation.org/for-patients/women-and-lc/.

[3] "Lung Cancer Among People Who Never Smoked," U.S. Centers for Disease Control and Prevention, December 4, 2023, https://www.cdc.gov/lung-cancer/nonsmokers/index.html#:_:text=cancer%2C%20and%20asbestos.-,In%20the%20United%20States%2C%20about%2010%25%20to%2020%25%20of,2%2C900%20of%20these%20lung%20cancers.

Professor of Medicine, Albert Einstein College of Medicine; Adjunct Professor of Medicine, Johns Hopkins University School of Medicine;

- Michelle Whitten, President, CEO, and Co-Founder, Global Down Syndrome Foundation;
- Randy Strozyk, President, American Ambulance Association; and,
- Christina Annunziata, MD, PhD, Senior Vice President of Extramural Discovery Science, American Cancer Society.

On May 16, 2024, the Subcommittee on Health met in open markup session and forwarded H.R. 4534, as amended, to the full Committee by a record vote of 21 yeas to 0 nays.

On June 12, 2024, the full Committee on Energy and Commerce met in open markup session and ordered H.R. 4534, as amended, favorably reported to the House by a record vote of 44 yeas and 0 nays.

Committee Votes

Clause 3(b) of rule XIII requires the Committee to list the record votes on the motion to report legislation and amendments thereto. The following reflects the record votes taken during the Committee consideration:

COMMITTEE ON ENERGY AND COMMERCE
118TH CONGRESS
ROLL CALL VOTE # 3

BILL: H.R. 4534, Women and Lung Cancer Research and Preventative Services Act of 2023

AMENDMENT: A motion by Chair Rodgers to order H.R. 4534 favorably reported to the House, as amended (Final Passage).

DISPOSITION: AGREED TO, by a recorded vote of 44 Yeas to 0 Nays.

REPRESENTATIVE	YEAS	NAYS	PRESENT	REPRESENTATIVE	YEAS	NAYS	PRESENT
Rep. Rodgers	X			Rep. Pallone	X		
Rep. Burgess	X			Rep. Eshoo	X		
Rep. Latta	X			Rep. DeGette	X		
Rep. Guthrie	X			Rep. Schakowsky	X		
Rep. Griffith	X			Rep. Matsui	X		
Rep. Bilirakis	X			Rep. Castor	X		
Rep. Bucshon	X			Rep. Sarbanes	X		

Rep. Hudson				Rep. Tonko	X		
Rep. Walberg				Rep. Clarke	X		
Rep. Carter	X			Rep. Cárdenas	X		
Rep. Duncan	X			Rep. Ruiz	X		
Rep. Palmer	X			Rep. Peters	X		
Rep. Dunn				Rep. Dingell	X		
Rep. Curtis				Rep. Veasey	X		
Rep. Lesko	X			Rep. Kuster	X		
Rep. Pence	X			Rep. Kelly	X		
Rep. Crenshaw				Rep. Barragán	X		
Rep. Joyce	X			Rep. Blunt Rochester			
Rep. Armstrong				Rep. Soto	X		
Rep. Weber	X			Rep. Craig	X		
Rep. Allen	X			Rep. Schrier	X		
Rep. Balderson	X			Rep. Trahan	X		
Rep. Fulcher	X			Rep. Fletcher	X		
Rep. Pfluger							
Rep. Harshbarger	X						
Rep. Miller-Meeks	X						
Rep. Cammack	X						
Rep. Obernolte	X						
Rep. James	X						

06/12/2024

Oversight Findings and Recommendations

Pursuant to clause 2(b)(1) of rule X and clause 3(c)(1) of rule XIII, the Committee held a hearing and made findings that are reflected in this report.

New Budget Authority, Entitlement Authority, and Tax Expenditures

Pursuant to clause 3(c)(2) of rule XIII, the Committee finds that H.R. 4534 would result in no new or increased budget authority, entitlement authority, or tax expenditures or revenues.

Congressional Budget Office Estimate

Pursuant to clause 3(c)(3) of rule XIII, at the time this report was filed, the cost estimate prepared by the Director of the Congressional Budget Office pursuant to section 402 of the Congressional Budget Act of 1974 was not available.

Federal Mandates Statement

The Committee adopts as its own the estimate of Federal mandates prepared by the Director of the Congressional Budget Office pursuant to section 423 of the Unfunded Mandates Reform Act.

Statement of General Performance Goals and Objectives

Pursuant to clause 3(c)(4) of rule XIII, the general performance goal or objective of this legislation is to review, evaluate the status of, and identify research and educational opportunities related to lung cancer in women and certain underserved populations.

Duplication of Federal Programs

Pursuant to clause 3(c)(5) of rule XIII, no provision of H.R. 4534 is known to be duplicative of another Federal program, including any program that was included in a report to Congress pursuant to section 21 of Public Law 111–139 or the most recent Catalog of Federal Domestic Assistance.

Related Committee and Subcommittee Hearings

Pursuant to clause 3(c)(6) of rule XIII, the following related hearing was used to develop or consider H.R. 4534:

- On February 14, 2024, the Subcommittee on Health held a hearing on H.R. 4534. The title of the hearing was "Legislative Proposals to

Support Patients and Caregivers." The Subcommittee received testimony from:

- Andy Shih, PhD, Chief Science Officer, Autism Speaks;
- Corey Feist, JD, MBA, Co-Founder and CEO, Dr. Lorna Breen Heroes' Foundation;
- Joanne Pike, DrPH, President and CEO, Alzheimer's Association;
- Gordon Tomaselli, MD, Former President, American Heart Association; Marilyn and Stanley M. Katz Dean, Emeritus and Professor of Medicine, Albert Einstein College of Medicine; Adjunct Professor of Medicine, Johns Hopkins University School of Medicine;
- Michelle Whitten, President, CEO, and Co-Founder, Global Down Syndrome Foundation;
- Randy Strozyk, President, American Ambulance Assciation; and,
- Christina Annunziata, MD, PhD, Senior Vice President of Extramural Discovery Science, American Cancer Society.

Committee Cost Estimate

Pursuant to clause 3(d)(1) of rule XIII, the Committee adopts as its own the cost estimate prepared by the Director of the Congressional Budget Office pursuant to section 402 of the Congressional Budget Act of 1974. At the time this report was filed, the estimate was not available.

Earmark, Limited Tax Benefits, and Limited Tariff Benefits

Pursuant to clause 9(e), 9(f), and 9(g) of rule XXI, the Committee finds that H.R. 4534 contains no earmarks, limited tax benefits, or limited tariff benefits.

Advisory Committee Statement

No advisory committees within the meaning of section 5(b) of the Federal Advisory Committee Act were created by this legislation.

Applicability to Legislative Branch

The Committee finds that the legislation does not relate to the terms and conditions of employment or access to public services or accommodations within the meaning of section 102(b)(3) of the Congressional Accountability Act.

Section-by-Section Analysis of the Legislation

Section 1. Short title

Section 1 provides that the Act may be cited as the "Women and Lung Cancer Research and Preventative Services Act of 2024."

Section 2. Interagency review to evaluate and identify opportunities for the acceleration of research on lung cancer in women and underserved populations, greater access to preventative services, and strategic public awareness and education campaigns.

Section 2 requires the Department of Health and Human Services (HHS) to conduct an interagency review on the status of, and identify research and education opportunities related to, women and certain underserved populations with lung cancer. The review would include assessments of current research and access to prevention services, the availability of research opportunities regarding prevention, detection, and treatment, and recommendations for national public education and screening strategies. This section also requires the HHS Secretary to submit a report to Congress detailing the results of the review within two years of enactment.

Changes in Existing Law Made by the Bill, as Reported

This legislation does not amend any existing Federal statute.

Chapter 10

Breast Cancer: Why the Environment Matters*

National Institutes of Health

A woman has a 1 in 8 chance of developing breast cancer in her lifetime, according to the American Cancer Society.

It is the second most common cancer among women in the United States, next to skin cancer. Breast cancer occurs mostly in women who are 50 years old or older.

Prevention Is Key

Supported by the National Institute of Environmental Health Sciences (NIEHS) and the National Cancer Institute (NCI), the Interagency Breast Cancer and Environmental Research Coordinating Committee concluded, in a landmark report1, that prevention is key to reducing the emotional, physical, and financial burden of breast cancer.

Research shows, in general, maintaining a healthy weight in adulthood, staying physically active, decreasing alcohol consumption, and consuming a nutritious diet can reduce the chance of developing cancer over your lifetime.

What Causes Breast Cancer?

Most women who develop breast cancer have no family history of the disease, suggesting an environmental link.

* This is an edited, reformatted and augmented version of National Institutes of Health, U.S. Department of Health and Human Services Publication, dated August 2023.

In: Understanding Cancer
Editor: Angela C. Ray
ISBN: 979-8-89530-769-4

In a study, inherited factors, such as the BRCA[1] or BRCA2 genes, accounted for only 27% of breast cancer risk.[2]

Although we know of many risk factors that increase women's chances of developing breast cancer, scientists do not completely understand what causes normal cells to become cancerous.

But most experts agree that a combination of genetic, hormonal, and environmental factors leads to breast cancer.

THE 20TH ANNIVERSARY

SISTER STUDY

BREAST CANCER RESEARCH

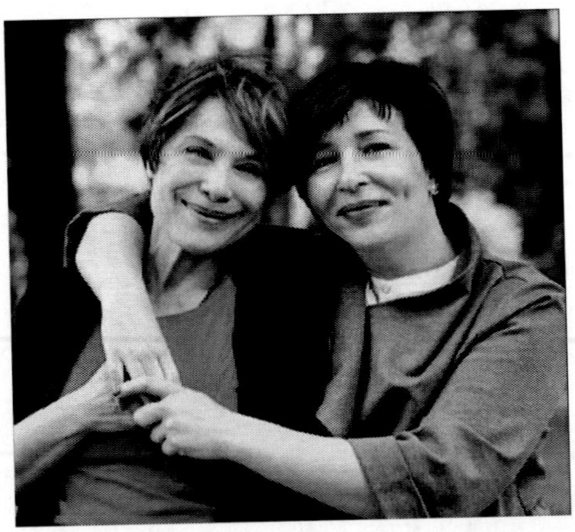

1 Interagency Breast Cancer and Environmental Research Coordinating Committee. 2013. Breast Cancer and the Environment: Prioritizing Prevention. Available: https://www.niehs.nih.gov/about/assets/docs/ibcercc_full_508.pdf.

2 Lichtenstein P, et al. 2000. Environmental and Heritable Factors in the Causation of Cancer: Analyses of Cohorts of Twins from Sweden, Denmark, and Finland. N Engl J Med 343(2):78-85.

What Does NIEHS Research Tell Us About Breast Cancer?

NIEHS plays a leadership role in funding and conducting studies on the ways in which genetic and environmental factors may affect breast cancer risk. For example, NIEHS scientists discovered women living in areas with higher levels of air pollution may have a higher risk of breast cancer.[3] Research can help determine environmental exposures that are linked to breast cancer.

Then, reducing those exposures may help prevent disease.

The Sister Study

The NIEHS Sister Study includes more than 50,000 sisters of women with breast cancer from the U.S., including Puerto Rico. The study looks at lifestyle and environmental exposures, as well as genetic and biological factors that may affect a woman's chance of developing breast cancer. Women with sisters who had breast cancer may have genetic profiles that make them twice as likely to develop breast cancer themselves. The study design offers the ability to identify environmental exposures over the life course that increase the chance of developing breast cancer, and to identify how genes and the environment interact to increase risk.

The Sister Study commemorates its 20th anniversary in 2023. Some important study findings are described in the following pages.

> "Sisters share many things including genes and early- life environments. By studying these sisters, we have increased the ability to detect health risks that are related to both the environment and genes. Over 20 years, we've conducted a wide range of research on breast cancer and also other diseases that are important for women."
> – Dale Sandler, Ph.D.,
> principal investigator of the NIEHS Sister Study

[3] Niehoff NM, et al. 2020. Outdoor air pollution and terminal duct lobular involution of the normal breast. Breast Cancer Res. 24;22(1):100.

Findings from the Sister Study

A wealth of data on exposures, including biological samples, allows the team to address many questions relating to factors associated with disease. In addition to breast cancer, the Sister Study has discovered other important information related to women's health. Key findings from this study are grouped around major themes.

Air Pollution

Air pollution is a complex mixture of many chemicals, including toxic metals, which can act as carcinogens. Air pollution has been linked to several diseases, such as cardiovascular disease, but less is known about its role in breast cancer.

Sister Study researchers found that higher levels of nitrogen dioxide (NO2), a component of air pollution related to traffic, was associated with increased breast cancer risk.[4] Radon gas, which occurs naturally in the environment, can break down into radioactive particles that can mix with air pollutants. Researchers found that exposure to these airborne radioactive particles was associated with a higher risk of estrogen receptor-negative breast cancer.[5]

Women who live in areas of air pollution with higher levels of lead, mercury, and cadmium have a greater chance of developing postmenopausal breast cancer.[6] Researchers evaluated whether dioxin may be associated with breast cancer risk. Publicly available data on industrial emissions at facilities located near participants' homes were used to estimate dioxin exposure levels. They found that long-term exposure to airborne dioxin emissions within 2 miles of participants' residences was associated with increased breast cancer risk. This association was strongest for emissions from municipal solid waste facilities. This finding indicates that living in proximity to industrial emissions may be linked to higher breast cancer rates.[7]

---

[4] White AJ, et al. 2019. Air Pollution, Clustering of Particulate Matter Components, and Breast Cancer in the Sister Study: A U.S.-Wide Cohort. Environ Health Perspect 127(10):107002.

[5] White AJ, et al. 2022. Exposure to particle radioactivity and breast cancer risk in the Sister Study: A U.S.-wide prospective cohort. Environ Health Perspect 130(4):47701.

[6] White AJ, et al. 2019. Metallic air pollutants and breast cancer risk in a nationwide cohort study. Epidemiology 30(1):20-8.

[7] Rhee J, et al. 2023. Residential proximity to dioxin emissions and risk of breast cancer in the sister study cohort. Environ Res 222:115297.

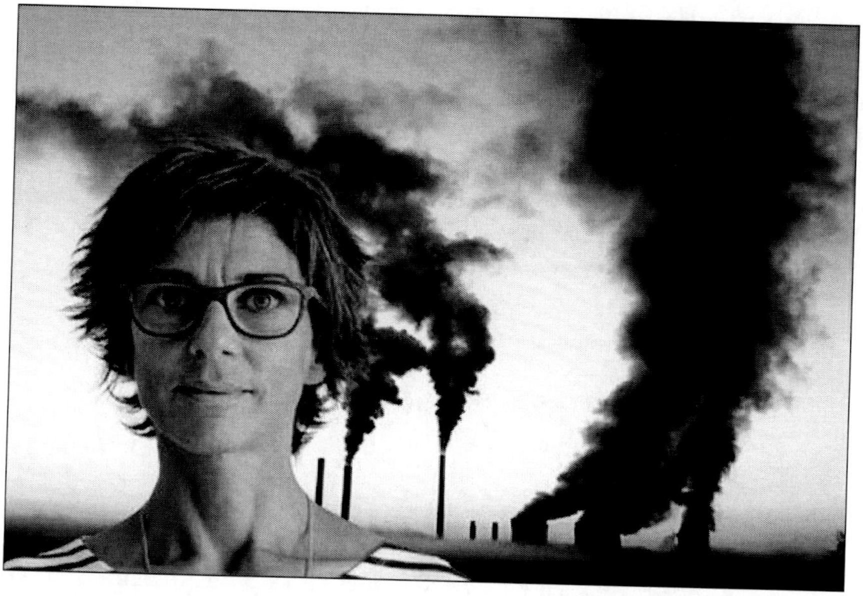

Diabetes

Pregnancy. Sister Study researchers found that developing diabetes during pregnancy, especially multiple pregnancies, increases the risk of type 2 diabetes later in life.[8]

Metformin use. While no association between type 2 diabetes and risk of developing estrogen receptor-positive breast cancer was found, there was a small increase in estrogen receptor- negative and triple-negative breast cancer among those with type 2 diabetes. Most women in the study with type 2 diabetes took metformin, a medication widely used to treat type 2 diabetes. These results support the hypothesis that even if type 2 diabetes is associated with increased breast cancer risk overall, metformin may help reduce the risk of developing estrogen receptor-positive breast cancer.[9]

[8] Diaz-Santana MV, et al. 2022. Persistence of risk for type 2 diabetes after gestational diabetes mellitus. Diabetes Care; doi:10.2337/dc21-1430.

[9] Park YM, et al. 2021. A prospective study of type 2 diabetes, metformin use, and risk of breast cancer. Ann Oncol 32(3):351-359.

Diet and Vitamin D

Sister Study research also works to identify the role of individual nutrients, particularly vitamin D, in breast cancer risk.

Among women who identified as Black/African American or non-Black Hispanic/Latina, those with low blood levels of vitamin D were more likely to develop breast cancer than women with adequate levels. These findings, along with prior studies, suggest that adequate vitamin D may be associated with a reduced chance of breast cancer.[10] Women who regularly took vitamin D supplements had lower rates of postmenopausal breast cancer.[11]

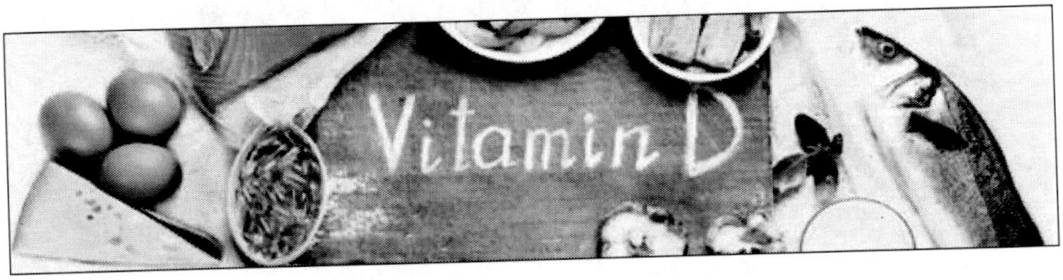

Genes and DNA Modifications

Genetics. Breast cancer genetic risk often refers to how the genes a woman is born with can influence her chance of getting breast cancer. However, as researchers showed, breast cancer may also be affected by naturally occurring changes to DNA, known as methylation, that occur after birth.[12] Women who developed breast cancer after joining the study were more likely to have changes in DNA methylation than those who did not have breast cancer, as seen in blood samples collected for the study.

Predicting risk. Sister Study researchers developed a new risk prediction score that may improve how women who are at higher risk for developing breast cancer can be identified.

This risk score is based on individual changes to DNA methylation associated with breast cancer risk, as well as multiple DNA methylation clocks

---

[10] O'Brien KM, et al. 2022. Vitamin D concentrations and breast cancer incidence among Black/African American and non-Black Hispanic/Latina women. Cancer 128(13):2463-2473.

[11] O'Brien KM, et al. 2017. Serum Vitamin D and Risk of Breast Cancer Within Five Years. Environ Health Perspect 125(7):077004.

[12] Xu Z, et al. 2020. Blood DNA Methylation and Breast Cancer: A Prospective Case-Cohort Analysis in the Sister Study. J Natl Cancer Inst 112(1):87-94.

associated with aging, morbidity and mortality risks, as well as breast cancer. Though this method returned promising results, further investigation and replication is needed to see if it will be useful in a clinical setting.[13]

Biological age. Chronological age is a leading risk factor for breast cancer. NIEHS scientists found that measures of biological aging based on combinations of DNA methylation changes, known as methylation-age clocks, may be tied to environmental exposures and the likelihood of developing breast cancer.[14]

The researchers later found that women who received breast cancer treatment, particularly radiation therapy, were biologically older than women who were never diagnosed with breast cancer.[15]

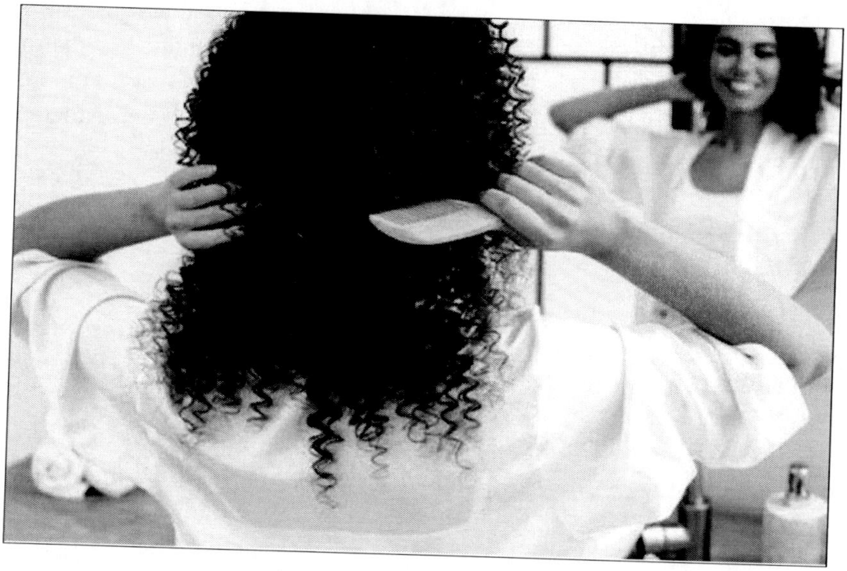

Hair Products

The potential for long-term health effects from certain chemicals in hair products are an interest area for Sister Study researchers.

---

[13] Kresovich JK, et al. 2022. Blood DNA methylation profiles improve breast cancer prediction. Mol Oncol 16(1):42-53.

[14] Kresovich JK, et al. 2019. Methylation-based biological age and breast cancer risk. J Natl Cancer Inst 111(10):1051-8.

[15] Kresovich JK, et al. 2023. Changes in methylation-based aging in women who do and do not develop breast cancer. J Natl Cancer Inst djad117.

Women who regularly used hair straighteners and dye were 9% more likely than women who did not to develop breast cancer. Among Black women, using permanent dyes every five to eight weeks or more was associated with a 60% increased chance of developing breast cancer, as compared with an 8% increased risk for white women.[16]

Researchers looked at hair product use during adolescence and found that frequent use of straighteners and perms may be associated with increased breast cancer risk later in life, particularly prior to menopause. This research suggests that some chemicals in such products may be harmful to health, even when used decades before.[17]

Other cancers. Frequent use of hair straighteners or relaxers (four or more times per year) was associated with twice the risk of ovarian cancer compared to non-users.[18] An association with uterine cancer was also found for women who frequently used chemical hair straightening products. But no associations between uterine cancer and use of hair dyes, bleach, highlights, or perms were found.[19] These findings are particularly relevant for Black/African American women who are more likely to use certain types of hair products.

Obesity

Women who were overweight or obese and had one or more metabolic abnormalities (such as elevated triglycerides, high blood sugar, or high blood pressure) had increased risk of postmenopausal breast cancer, as did overweight or obese women with no metabolic abnormalities. Risk of postmenopausal breast cancer was also higher in women with normal weight, but high measures of obesity in the mid-section of their bodies.[20]

---

[16] Eberle CE, et al. 2019. Hair dye and chemical straightener use and breast cancer risk in a large US population of black and white women. Int J Cancer 147(2):383-391.

[17] White AJ, et al. 2021. Adolescent use of hair dyes, straighteners and perms in relation to breast cancer risk. Int J Cancer 148(9):2255-63.

[18] White AJ, et al. 2021. Use of hair products in relation to ovarian cancer risk. Carcinogenesis 42(9):1189-95.

[19] Chang CJ, et al. 2022. Use of Straighteners and Other Hair Products and Incident Uterine Cancer. J Natl Cancer Inst 114(12):1636-1645.

[20] Park YM, et al. 2017. The association between metabolic health, obesity phenotype and the risk of breast cancer. Int J Cancer 140(12):2657-66.

Sleep

Nighttime light, from inside the bedroom or shining in from outside the residence, is thought to increase the risk of breast cancer by disrupting the body's natural 24-hour (circadian) rhythms, which serve a wide variety of biologic functions.

Sleeping with a television on, or at least one light on in the bedroom, was associated with a small (9%) increase in breast cancer risk.[21]

Trouble sleeping. Researchers also found trouble sleeping four or more nights per week was associated with increased breast cancer risk.[21]

Social and Early-Life Factors

Activity. Women who exercised or played sports more than seven hours a week during ages 5-19 had a lower risk of breast cancer as adults.[22]

Trauma. Sister Study participants were asked if they experienced certain traumatic experiences during childhood and adolescence, and about half disclosed at least one traumatic experience before age 18. Traumatic events may include sexual, physical, or emotional abuse, and financial hardships. Experiencing either sexual trauma and household dysfunction, or some other early-life trauma, was associated with greater risk of developing breast cancer. But breast cancer risk due to early- life trauma appeared lower among participants who reported constant childhood social support. This research suggests that different types of early-life traumatic experiences may contribute to breast cancer risk.[23]

Early development. Earlier age at the first menstrual period (menarche) is known to be associated with increased breast cancer risk. Sister Study researchers found that earlier age of breast development (thelarche) is also associated with breast cancer risk. Experiencing early menarche (before age 12) and early thelarche (before age 10) together was associated with a greater risk than either factor on its own.[24]

---

[21] White AJ, et al. 2017. Sleep characteristics, light at night and breast cancer risk in a prospective cohort. Int J Cancer 141(11):2204-2214.

[22] Neihoff NM, et al. 2017. Childhood and teenage physical activity and breast cancer risk. Breast Cancer Res Treat 164(3):697-705.

[23] Woo JMP, et al. 2022. Latent class models of early-life trauma and incident breast cancer. Epidemiology 33(5):729-38.

[24] Goldberg M, et al. 2020. Pubertal timing and breast cancer risk in the Sister Study cohort. Breast Cancer Res 22(1):112.

Future Direction for the Sister Study

The Sister Study collects more detailed information than many other studies, allowing researchers to ask and answer more complicated questions. They have been able, and will continue, to partner with researchers all over the world.

Participants in the study are diverse, which allows researchers to study health disparities and the health effects of factors related to where someone lives.

A newer challenge is to understand how changes in the climate may affect breast cancer risk. For example, the researchers are studying the effects of heat and how stressors from experiencing natural disasters may relate to breast cancer risk.

They also are focusing more on the ways that environmental factors may affect how well women fare after diagnosis and treatment for breast cancer.

To learn more about the NIEHS Sister Study, visit https://sisterstudy.niehs.nih.gov/English/index1.htm.

Two Sister Study

A related NIEHS study focuses on women under 50 with young-onset breast cancer and their sisters without breast cancer. This study found certain factors may reduce the risk of young-onset breast cancer, such as older age at menarche, younger age at menopause, premenopausal hysterectomy, and early age at first-term pregnancy.[25]

Other NIEHS-Funded Research

NIEHS, along with the NCI, studied developmental periods in women's lifespans, such as puberty, pregnancy, and menopause, to identify factors related to breast cancer.

As a result, future prevention efforts may be targeted and more effective. Findings include:

---

25 O'Brien KM, et al. 2015. Risk factors for young-onset invasive and in situ breast cancer. Cancer Causes Control. 26(12):1771-8.

- Exposures to common chemicals may change the timing of puberty. For example, girls exposed to high levels of triclosan, used in some antimicrobial soaps, had early breast development. Also, girls exposed to high levels of benzophenone-3, found in some sunscreens, had later breast development.[26]
- The chance of developing breast cancer may increase with exposure to endocrine-disrupting chemicals during these periods: prenatal development, puberty, pregnancy, and menopausal transition.[27]
- About 300 chemicals used in personal care products, flame retardants, food processing, pesticides, and other purposes were tested using in vitro assays and found to affect hormones known to increase breast cancer risk. [28]

NIEHS continues to fund grants for breast cancer research. For example, grant recipients are studying:

- Why African American women are more likely to get aggressive forms of breast cancer than other women.
- How disrupting a woman's biological clock or circadian rhythm (through shift work or time zone changes, for example) can affect the risk of developing breast cancer.
- How chemicals like PFAS may affect the chance of developing breast cancer.

National Toxicology Program (NTP)

An interagency program headquartered at NIEHS, NTP lists six substances in the Report on Carcinogens because they cause or may cause breast cancer in humans: diethylstilbestrol (DES), a synthetic estrogen that was used to prevent miscarriages; steroidal estrogens used for menopausal therapy; X-ray and

---

[26] Wolff MS, et al. 2015. Breast Cancer and Environment Research Program. 2016. Environmental phenols and pubertal development in girls. Environ Int 84:174-180.

[27] Terry MB, et al. 2019. Environmental exposures during windows of susceptibility for breast cancer: a framework for prevention research. Breast Cancer Research; doi: 10.1186/s13058-019-1168-2.

[28] Cardona B, Rudel RA. 2021. Application of an in Vitro Assay to Identify Chemicals That Increase Estradiol and Progesterone Synthesis and Are Potential Breast Cancer Risk Factors. Environ Health Perspect. 129(7):77003.

gamma radiation; alcoholic beverages; tobacco smoking; and ethylene oxide, a sterilizing agent.[29]

After conducting cancer assessments for working at night, NTP found that persistent night shift work that disrupts circadian rhythms can cause breast cancer in women. This type of work is considered frequent and long-term, especially beginning in early adulthood.[30]

For more information on the National Institute of Environmental Health Sciences, visit https://niehs.nih.gov.

---

29 National Toxicology Program. 15th RoC Dashboard. DOI: https://doi.org/10.22427/NTP-DATA-ROC-15 [accessed 17 July 2023].

30 National Toxicology Program. 2021. Cancer Hazard Assessment Report on Night Shift Work and Light at Night. Available: https://ntp.niehs.nih.gov/ntp/results/pubs/ cancer_assessment/lanfinal20210400_508.pdf.

Chapter 11

Pediatric Cancer Studies: Early Results of the Research to Accelerate Cures and Equity for Children Act*

U.S. Covernment Accountability Office

Chair
Ranking Member
Committee on Health, Education, Labor, and Pensions
United States Senate

The Honorable Cathy McMorris Rodgers
Chair

The Honorable Frank Pallone, Jr.
Ranking Member
Committee on Energy and Commerce
House of Representatives

Pediatric cancer is the leading cause of death by disease past infancy among children from birth to age 14 in the United States, according to the National Cancer Institute. The National Cancer Institute estimated that in 2022 alone, 10,470 new cases of cancer would be diagnosed in children—of those, around 10 percent are expected to ultimately die from the disease.[1] While survival rates for pediatric cancers more broadly have improved over the last few

---

* This is an edited, reformatted and augmented version of the United States Government Accountability Office Report, Publication No., GAO-23-105947, dated January 31, 2023.

[1] National Cancer Institute, "Childhood Cancers" (Aug. 19, 2022), accessed Nov. 2, 2022, https://www.cancer.gov/types/childhood-cancers.

In: Understanding Cancer
Editor: Angela C. Ray
ISBN: 979-8-89530-769-4

decades, survival rates for some pediatric cancers remain low. For example, the National Cancer Institute reports that only 10 percent of children with diffuse intrinsic pontine glioma, a rare brain tumor, survive 2 years after being diagnosed.

There have been relatively few drugs approved to treat pediatric cancer. As of December 2022, there were 54 drugs approved to treat pediatric cancer.[2] As a result, clinicians treating pediatric patients have limited options. Clinicians may opt to use a cancer drug approved for adults; however, in these instances, there may be limited available information specific to the safety and effectiveness of the drug in the pediatric population, according to Food and Drug Administration (FDA) officials.[3]

Pediatric Cancers

Pediatric oncologists often note that children are not just little adults. Children are less likely to suffer from some common adult cancers like lung, breast, colon, and prostate cancer.

Instead, the most common cancers among pediatric patients are brain and central nervous system cancers, leukemia (blood cancers), and Hodgkin and non-Hodgkin lymphomas (lymphatic cancers).

- Brain and central nervous system cancers. The growth of abnormal cells in brain tissue and central nervous system.
- Leukemia. Cancer that starts in blood-forming tissue, such as the bone marrow, and causes large numbers of abnormal blood cells to be produced and enter the bloodstream.
- Lymphoma. Comprised of two basic categories—Hodgkin and non-Hodgkin lymphomas, these are cancers that begin in the cells of the immune system.

Source: GAO summary of information from the National Cancer Institute. I GAO-23-105947.

---

[2] Food and Drug Administration, "Pediatric Oncology Drug Approvals" (Dec. 2022), accessed Jan. 18, 2023, https://www.fda.gov/about-fda/oncology-center-excellence/pediatric-oncology-drug-approvals.

[3] Unapproved use of an FDA-approved drug is often called "off-label" use. Food and Drug Administration, "Understanding Unapproved Use of Approved Drugs 'Off Label'," (Feb. 5, 2018), accessed Dec. 6, 2022, https://www.fda.gov/patients/learn-about-expanded-access-and-other-treatment-options/understanding-unapproved-use-approved-drugs-label. FDA officials noted that much of the pediatric cancer standard of care management includes use of cancer drugs not specifically approved for use in children.

Since 2003, to encourage research into pediatric treatments, sponsors of certain adult drugs and biologics (we refer to both as drugs in this report) have been required to conduct pediatric studies as part of the drug approval process per the Pediatric Research Equity Act of 2003.[4] However, this requirement has frequently been waived for sponsors of adult cancer drugs, because adults and children typically get different types of cancer.[5] For example, FDA would not have required a sponsor to conduct a pediatric study for a prostate cancer drug, because prostate cancer generally does not occur in children.

In more recent years, researchers have improved their understanding of cancers and are developing drugs that target the disease at the molecular level—referred to as molecularly targeted drugs.[6] With this approach, a drug that targets a molecular abnormality found in both adult and pediatric cancers can potentially be used to treat both populations, although their cancer types may differ.

Recognizing the potential of molecularly targeted drugs and to facilitate the development of new, safe, and effective drugs to treat children, Congress passed, and the President signed into law, the FDA Reauthorization Act of 2017, to include a provision commonly known as the Research to Accelerate Cures and Equity for Children Act (RACE Act).[7] Specifically, as of August 18, 2020, the RACE Act requires drug sponsors that intend to apply for approval of molecularly targeted adult cancer drugs to submit their planned approach for studying the drug in the pediatric population (referred to as an initial pediatric study plan).[8] The RACE Act requirement also applies to

---

[4] The National Cancer Institute defines a biologic drug as a substance that is made from a living organism or its products, and is used in the prevention, diagnosis, or treatment of cancer and other diseases. A sponsor means a person who takes responsibility for and initiates a clinical investigation. The sponsor may be an individual or pharmaceutical company, governmental agency, academic institution, private organization, or other organization.

[5] Under the Pediatric Research Equity Act of 2003, applications for new active ingredients, indications, dosage forms, dosing regimens, or routes of administration are generally required to include pediatric studies. FDA may grant a full or partial waiver of this requirement if certain conditions are met—for example, if the product is intended to treat a disease or condition that does not occur in a pediatric population. See 21 U.S.C. § 355c(a)(1)(A), (a)(2), and (a)(5). For our prior work on this act, see GAO, *Pediatric Research: Products Studied under Two Related Laws, but Improved Tracking Needed by FDA*, GAO-11-457 (Washington, D.C.: May 31, 2011).

[6] In this process, researchers first identify molecular targets associated with the cancer—for example, some proteins may be present in cancerous cells but not in non-cancerous cells. Then, researchers develop a drug that binds or interacts with the molecular target, thereby slowing or stopping the progression of cancer cell growth.

[7] Pub. L. No. 115-52, § 504, 131 Stat. 1005, 1039-46 (codified at 21 U.S.C. § 355c).

[8] RACE Act studies are generally required for original applications for new active ingredients if the drug is intended to treat an adult cancer and directed at a molecular target that is

molecularly targeted adult cancer drugs that qualify as orphan drugs—generally, drugs intended to treat a disease or condition that affects fewer than 200,000 people in the U.S.

The FDA Reauthorization Act of 2017 includes a provision for GAO to review the effectiveness of the pediatric study requirements enacted by the RACE Act.[9] In this report, we describe the effects of the act.

To describe the effects of the RACE Act, we reviewed data provided by FDA officials on new molecularly targeted adult cancer drugs with initial pediatric study plans for the period from the implementation of the RACE Act requirement (August 18, 2020), through August 18, 2022.

These data describe the 85 initial pediatric study plans that FDA received, reviewed, and agreed to during this time period.[10] We used these data to determine the number of pediatric cancer studies sponsors planned to conduct and the number expected to receive waivers, among other information. We assessed the reliability of these data by comparing them to information in other sources, such as FDA drug approval letters and an April 2022 FDA report to Congress; interviewing knowledgeable agency officials about the data; and performing checks of the data for accuracy and completeness.[11] Based on these steps, we found these data to be reliable for the purposes of our reporting objective.

Additionally, to learn more about the effects of the RACE Act, we conducted interviews with FDA officials and a judgmentally selected sample of 14 non-federal stakeholders. To capture a broad range of perspectives, including those of the drug industry and patients, we selected and interviewed individuals from four patient advocacy groups, two industry groups, and five drug sponsors, as well as three pediatric cancer researchers. The views of the 14 stakeholders are not generalizable; however, they provide insights on the effects of the RACE Act, including related benefits and challenges experienced since its implementation.

We conducted this performance audit from March 2022 through January 2023 in accordance with generally accepted government auditing standards.

---

substantially relevant to the growth or progression of a pediatric cancer. FDA may grant a full or partial waiver of this requirement if certain conditions are met. See 21U.S.C. §355c(a)(1)(B), (a)(3), and (a)(5).

[9] Pub. L. No. 115-52. § 504(f), 131 Stat. at 1045-46.

[10] FDA received and agreed upon at least two additional pediatric study plans prior to implementation of the RACE Act requirement. According to FDA officials, these plans were submitted by sponsors in anticipation of the RACE Act requirement.

[11] Food and Drug Administration, *Best Pharmaceuticals for Children Act and Pediatric Research Equity Act Status Report to Congress July 1, 2015–June 30, 2020* (Apr. 21, 2022).

Those standards require that we plan and perform the audit to obtain sufficient, appropriate evidence to provide a reasonable basis for our findings and conclusions based on our audit objectives. We believe that the evidence obtained provides a reasonable basis for our findings and conclusions based on our audit objective.

Background

FDA guidance encourages sponsors of adult molecularly targeted cancer drugs to meet with the agency early in the clinical study process to discuss their initial pediatric study plans.[12] The required components of an initial pediatric study plan include

- an outline of the pediatric study or studies that the sponsor plans to conduct (including, to the extent practicable, study objectives and design, age groups, relevant endpoints— the result measured to determine effectiveness—and statistical approach);
- any request for a full waiver, partial waiver, or deferral along with supporting justification; and
- other information specified in the regulations issued by FDA.[13]

In some cases, a sponsor may believe that a pediatric study is not warranted or is not suitable for some pediatric age groups. These sponsors can

[12] Sponsors are required to submit their initial pediatric study plan to FDA for review no later than 60 calendar days after the date of the end-of-phase 2 meeting, or at another time as agreed upon between FDA and the sponsor. The purpose of the end-of-phase 2 meetings is to determine the safety of proceeding to phase 3 clinical trials, to evaluate the phase 3 plan and protocols and the adequacy of current studies and plans to assess pediatric safety and effectiveness, and to identify any additional information necessary to support a marketing application for the uses under investigation.

[13] See 21 U.S.C. § 355c(e)(2)(B). FDA guidance also notes that, in certain situations, it may be premature to include a detailed outline of a planned pediatric study (or studies) because additional data are needed. In these instances, the outline of the pediatric studies should include a brief explanation for the lack of more detailed information. Examples of other information that FDA recommends be included in such plans are a timeline for the pediatric development plan and agreements for pediatric studies with other regulatory agencies (for example, FDA's European counterpart, the European Medicines Agency) when available. Food and Drug Administration, Center for Drug Evaluation and Research and Center for Biologics Evaluation and Research, *Pediatric Study Plans: Content of and Process for Submitting Initial Pediatric Study Plans and Amended Initial Pediatric Study Plans, Guidance for Industry* (July 2020).

use their initial pediatric study plan to request that FDA waive their pediatric study requirements entirely (referred to as a full waiver) or waive the pediatric study requirements for some age groups (referred to as a partial waiver). Sponsors with required pediatric studies may also request permission to submit the reports of studies after the adult drug is approved—these are referred to as deferrals. Deferred pediatric studies then become postmarketing requirements—studies that a sponsor completes after FDA has approved a product for marketing.[14]

The required pediatric studies under the RACE Act are not necessarily designed to provide sufficient safety and effectiveness information for drug approval. RACE Act studies are designed to yield clinically meaningful pediatric study data about the drug's safety, dosing, and preliminary efficacy to inform potential pediatric uses of the drug. Depending on the results of a RACE Act study, FDA may choose to issue a written request to a sponsor to conduct additional pediatric studies, which may lead to eventual drug approval, if the drug is shown to be safe and effective in the pediatric population.[15] Sponsor completion of those additional study requests is voluntary. See figure 1 for an illustration of the drug development timeline and process with a pediatric study.

---

[14] FDA reviews requests for a full waiver, partial waiver, or deferral in the initial pediatric study plan and makes a recommendation as to whether the request meets statutory criteria when it agrees to the plan. FDA does not finalize its decision on any request for a waiver or deferral until it approves the drug for use in adults.

[15] Before FDA can approve a drug, the sponsor must provide evidence to demonstrate the drug is safe and effective for its intended use. According to FDA officials, in some cases, a sponsor's initial pediatric study plan has included plans for more definitive studies that may be sufficient for approval for use in the pediatric population. Agency officials noted that decisions related to approval are made following sufficient FDA review of the application.

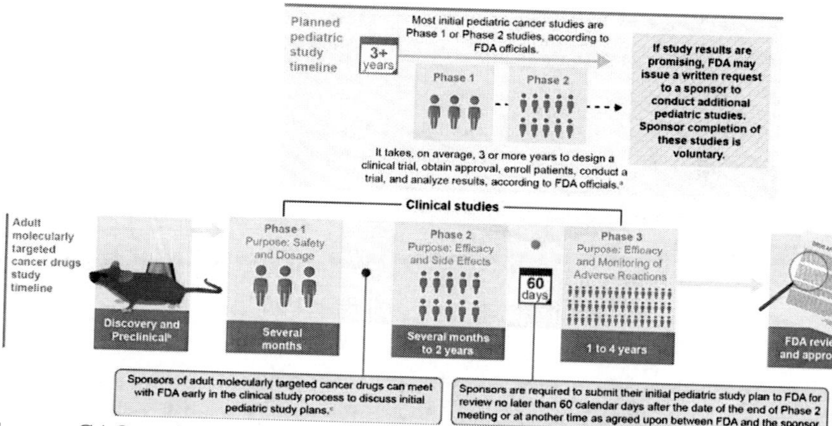

Source: GAO analysis of Food and Drug Administration (FDA) documentation and information provided by FDA officials. | GAO-23-105947.

Note: This figure provides an illustrative example and is not intended to represent the path or time frames taken by all drugs and initial pediatric study plans. In this figure, GAO refers to both drugs and biologics as drugs.

[a] According to FDA officials, this timeline will vary based on several factors, including the rarity of the cancer, whether the pediatric study is international, and sponsor resources.

[b] In the discovery and development phase (referred to in the figure as "discovery"), researchers identify a promising drug compound for development through new insights and then conduct experiments to gather information on the compound. In the preclinical phase, researchers study a drug's toxicity in a laboratory setting so they can determine whether the drug has the potential to cause serious harm prior to testing in people.

[c] An initial pediatric study plan is a document that outlines the planned approach to study a drug in a pediatric population, which may include a plan to request a study deferral or waiver. While FDA makes a recommendation on any request for a waiver or deferral in an initial pediatric study plan, FDA does not finalize its decision until it approves the drug for use in adults.

Figure 1. Illustrative Example of Drug Development Timeline and Process with a Pediatric Study.

The RACE Act Has Contributed to an Increase in Planned Pediatric Studies, but Long- Term Effects Are Unclear

The RACE Act Has Contributed to an Increase in the Number of Planned Pediatric Studies

The RACE Act has contributed to an increase in the number of pediatric studies that sponsors of molecularly targeted adult cancer drugs plan to conduct, according to data provided by FDA. Specifically, there have been 32 initial pediatric study plans submitted to FDA with intentions to conduct a pediatric study since the requirement was implemented on August 18, 2020, to August 18, 2022. Prior to the RACE Act, sponsors would not have been required to conduct most of these studies. This is either because (1) the drug has orphan status and would have been exempt from requirements to conduct a pediatric study or (2) the sponsor would have received a waiver, because the adult condition rarely or never occurs in children.[16]

Specifically, of the 32 planned pediatric studies, five are for drugs that FDA has approved and have postmarketing requirements for pediatric studies, according to FDA documentation. Pediatric studies would not have been required for any of the five approved drugs prior to RACE Act implementation. (See enclosure I for more information on the adult and pediatric indications and molecular targets associated with these five approved drugs.) The remaining 27 planned pediatric studies are for drugs still in development—most of these planned studies would not have been required pre-RACE Act. See table 1 for more information on the planned pediatric studies that would have been exempt due to the drug's orphan status or received an adult indication waiver prior to the RACE Act.

[16] Under the Pediatric Research Equity Act of 2003, which predates the RACE Act, requirements for pediatric studies do not apply to orphan drugs. See 21 U.S.C. § 355c(k)(1). However, under the RACE Act, orphan drugs that are molecularly targeted cancer drugs are not exempt from pediatric study requirements. See 21 U.S.C. § 355c(k)(2). FDA has maintained a list of adult conditions that rarely or never occur in pediatric patients, and prior to the RACE Act, drugs intended for these conditions received a pediatric study waiver, as pediatric studies for these conditions would be impossible or highly impracticable. See 21 U.S.C. § 355c(a)(5).

Orphan Drugs

Orphan drugs include drugs for diseases affecting fewer than 200,000 people in the United States or for which there is no reasonable expectation of recovering the cost of the drug development and marketing from U.S. sales. Prior to the Research to Accelerate Cures and Equity for Children Act (RACE Act), all adult orphan drugs were exempt from pediatric study requirements— meaning that they did not have to study the drug in pediatric populations.

Postmarketing Requirements Postmarketing requirements are studies that drug sponsors are required to conduct after FDA has approved a product for marketing. These studies provide additional information about the safety, efficacy, and optimal use of an approved drug.

Source: GAO summary of Food and Drug Administration (FDA) information. I GAO-23-105947.

Table 1. Planned pediatric studies under the RACE act that could have been required prior to RACE act implementation, August 18, 2020 through August 18, 2022

Drug approval status	Number of planned pediatric studies under RACE Act	Number of planned pediatric studies that would have received an exemption or waiver pre-RACE Act[a]	Number of planned pediatric studies that could have been required pre-RACE Act
Approved drugs	5	5[b]	0
Drugs in development	27	20[c]	7[d]
Total	32	25	7

Source: GAO analysis of data provided by Food and Drug Administration (FDA). | GAO-23-105947.

Note: The RACE Act, or Research to Accelerate Cures and Equity for Children Act, is the common name for a provision included in the FDA Reauthorization Act of 2017.

[a] Under the Pediatric Research Equity Act of 2003, which predates the RACE Act, requirements for pediatric studies do not apply to drugs for an indication for which orphan designation has been granted. See 21 U.S.C. § 355c(k)(1). These are commonly referred to as "orphan drugs." However, under the RACE Act, orphan drugs that are molecularly targeted cancer drugs are not exempt from pediatric study requirements. See 21 U.S.C. § 355c(k)(2). Orphan drugs are drugs that are

intended to treat diseases affecting fewer than 200,000 people in the United States or for which there is no reasonable expectation of recovering the cost of the drug development and marketing from U.S. sales. FDA has also maintained a list of adult indications that rarely or never occur in the pediatric population, and prior to the RACE Act, drugs intended for these conditions received a pediatric study waiver, as pediatric studies for these indications would be impossible or highly impracticable. See 21 U.S.C. § 355c(a)(5).

[b] Four of the five approved drugs have orphan status, and the other approved drug is for a condition that rarely or never occurs in the pediatric population, and for which a pediatric study would be impossible or highly impracticable.

[c] Seventeen of the 27 drugs in development have orphan status, and three of the 27 drugs in development are for a condition that rarely or never occurs in the pediatric population, and for which a pediatric study would be impossible or highly impracticable.

[d] FDA officials noted that it was highly likely the agency would have waived requirements to conduct a pediatric study for the majority of the seven drugs noted in this column due to the rarity of the indication being sought in pediatric patients.

While the RACE Act has contributed to an increase in the number of planned pediatric studies, not all sponsors of molecularly targeted adult cancer drugs will be required to complete pediatric studies. Specifically, since RACE Act implementation, sponsors have submitted 53 other pediatric study plans to FDA for which FDA and the sponsor have agreed with the sponsor's plan to request a full waiver—meaning that a pediatric study would not have to be conducted.[17]

Reasons for these waiver requests vary—for example, some sponsors requested waivers of the requirement because FDA and thc sponsor determined the drug does not represent a meaningful therapeutic benefit over existing therapies for children and is not likely to be used in a substantial number of children. For more information on full waivers and the waiver justifications, as well as information on planned pediatric studies with partial waivers or deferrals, see enclosure II.

---

[17] While FDA makes a recommendation on any request for a waiver or deferral in an initial pediatric study plan, FDA does not finalize its decision until it approves the drug for use in adults.

Long-Term Effects of RACE Act Are Not Yet Clear; FDA and Stakeholders Optimistic

It is too soon to know if the RACE Act will increase the number of drugs approved to treat pediatric cancers. This is because, according to FDA officials, the planned studies are still in the early phases or have not yet begun, so the final study outcomes, including whether they show promise in pediatric populations, are not yet known. These studies will take years to complete given the long timelines associated with pediatric drug development. For example, it will be at least 3 years before the first of the required pediatric studies for already approved adult drugs is completed and the associated reports are submitted to FDA, according to drug approval letters.

Additionally, because RACE Act studies are designed to yield clinically meaningful pediatric study data about the drug's safety, dosing, and preliminary efficacy to inform potential pediatric uses of the drug, FDA officials told us that additional studies may be needed for a drug to be approved for use in pediatric populations. These further studies are not required by the RACE Act. Instead, FDA may issue a written request to a sponsor to conduct additional pediatric studies.[18]

While the long-term effects of the RACE Act are not yet clear, FDA officials and nine stakeholders we interviewed including researchers, patient advocates, and drug sponsors told us they expect the RACE Act to have positive effects in furthering pediatric cancer research and drug development. For example, representatives from one drug sponsor we spoke with noted that since RACE Act implementation they have seen wider interest in pediatric cancer, which they view as a positive step. Officials with a research organization made similar comments, stating that they have received increased inquiries about conducting pediatric cancer studies.

This positive outlook was echoed by FDA officials, who told us they are optimistic that the RACE Act will increase the number of drugs available for pediatric patients with cancer.

[18] Sponsor completion of additional studies requested by FDA through a written request is voluntary. As an incentive, if a sponsor opts to conduct the requested studies, it can gain an additional 6 months of marketing exclusivity once the requested studies are completed, based on the terms outlined in FDA's written request. See 21 U.S.C. § 355a.

Patient Enrollment in Pediatric Studies Is Challenging; FDA Taking Steps to Address

Enrolling patients in pediatric cancer studies is a long-standing challenge due to limited patient populations. The increase in planned pediatric studies under the RACE Act could further exacerbate these enrollment challenges, according to FDA officials and six stakeholders we spoke with. Pediatric cancer, considered a rare disease, includes many subtypes of even more rare cancers. One researcher told us that the many different types and subtypes of pediatric cancers—each potentially needing its own study—can make potential patient population pools even narrower. Additionally, pediatric patients with cancer are often only enrolled in clinical studies when the existing cancer treatment fails or the patient has relapsed, further reducing the pool of potential enrollees, according FDA officials.

Because the patient population is so small, researchers may also face challenges finding study enrollees who are diverse and representative of the wider pediatric cancer population.

According to recent research, pediatric cancer clinical studies may not always be representative of a diverse population.[19] In April 2022, FDA published draft guidance that noted the importance of adequate representation of children from racial and ethnic minority backgrounds in pediatric clinical studies.[20]

Enrollment challenges have the potential to affect whether pediatric cancer studies are completed, and whether the data are sufficient to determine significant effects of the studied drug. Two researchers we spoke with expressed concerns that enrollment challenges could ultimately lead to pediatric studies not being completed.

FDA officials noted that they are prepared to work with sponsors to address enrollment challenges. FDA has taken steps intended to help address such challenges, including

---

[19] Paula Aristizabal et al., "Disparities in Pediatric Oncology: The 21st Century Opportunity to Improve Outcomes for Children and Adolescents with Cancer," *American Society of Clinical Oncology Educational Book*, vol. 41 (2021).

[20] Food and Drug Administration, *Diversity Plans to Improve Enrollment of Participants from Underrepresented Racial and Ethnic Populations in Clinical Trials Draft Guidance for Industry*, (Apr. 2022). GAO has also examined diversity in cancer clinical trials more broadly, see GAO, *Cancer Clinical Trials: Federal Actions and Selected Non-Federal Practices to Facilitate Diversity of Patients*, GAO-23-105245 (Washington, D.C.: Dec. 22, 2022).

- providing guidance on innovative study designs;
- coordinating with its European counterpart, the European Medicines Agency; and
- developing guidance on determining pediatric studies for similar drugs.

Providing guidance on innovative study designs. FDA's guidance for industry describes six innovative approaches sponsors may take to address small pediatric populations. For example, sponsors may be able to enroll pediatric patients in a cohort for an existing adult study, leveraging the resources of the adult study instead of opening up an entirely new clinical trial solely for pediatric patients.[21] FDA officials noted that several sponsors have included innovative study designs in their pediatric study plans. For example, FDA officials told us that there are initial pediatric study plans where the sponsor will study a drug or drug combination across multiple cancer populations, referred to as a basket trial. Basket trials minimize the number of patients needed for a clinical trial with a specific type of cancer, because researchers can draw from patient populations with multiple cancer types. A sponsor and an advocacy group we spoke with also noted the value of innovative study designs in overcoming enrollment challenges.

Coordinating with the European Medicines Agency. FDA guidance notes that coordination with its European counterpart—the European Medicines Agency, which has pediatric cancer study requirements that predate the RACE Act—can help prevent duplication of studies and competition for scarce pediatric patients with cancer. According to FDA officials, since RACE Act implementation, FDA and the European Medicines Agency have been working closely, including holding joint discussions regarding the scientific and clinical justification for pediatric studies of new adult cancer drugs, their feasibility given the limited patient populations, the appropriate timing of studies, and study designs and timelines.[22] The value of this coordination was echoed by drug sponsors. For example, two sponsors said cooperation between FDA and the European Medicines Agency was important and could

---

[21] Food and Drug Administration, FDARA Implementation Guidance for Pediatric Studies of Molecularly Targeted Oncology Drugs: Amendments to Sec. 505B of the FD&C Act. Guidance for Industry (May 2021).

[22] According to FDA guidance for industry, the European Medicines Agency and FDA work together to provide common commentary on some proposed pediatric study plans and also have a mechanism for formal parallel scientific advice from both agencies for some cancer drug applications. Food and Drug Administration, *FDARA Implementation Guidance for Pediatric Studies of Molecularly Targeted Oncology Drugs.*

potentially allow sponsors to fulfill both agencies' pediatric study requirements with a single study.

Developing guidance on determining pediatric studies for similar drugs. FDA officials told us that the agency is developing guidance for determining pediatric study requirements among multiple same-in-class drugs. These drugs have the same molecular target and are in the same pharmacologic class, meaning they function similarly to each other. Because pediatric studies of same-in-class drugs will draw from the same small patient pool, there are concerns that sponsors may struggle to enroll enough patients, according to FDA officials and four stakeholders we spoke with, including one researcher, one industry association, and two drug sponsors. Three sponsors and an industry association we spoke with noted that it is helpful in drug development planning to understand how FDA makes decisions regarding which same-in-class drugs require a pediatric study, and which will have their requirements waived. FDA officials told us the guidance will likely take a few years to develop and finalize, including time for public comment.[23]

Agency Comments

We provided a draft of this report to the Department of Health and Human Services (HHS) for review and comment. HHS provided technical comments, which we incorporated as appropriate. We are sending copies of this report to the appropriate congressional committees and the Secretary of Health and Human Services. In addition, the report will be available at no charge on the GAO website at http://www.gao.gov.

If you or your staff have any questions about this report, please contact me at (202) 512-7114 or DeniganMacauleyM@gao.gov. Contact points for our offices of Congressional Relations and Public Affairs may be found on the last page of this report. In addition to the contact named above, Deirdre Brown (Assistant Director), Luke Baron (Analyst-in-Charge), Maggie Baucom, and Meghann Lewis made key contributions to this report. Also contributing were Joycelyn Cudjoe, Kaitlin Farquharson, Ying Hu, Roxanna Sun, and Janet Wilson.

---

[23] In May 2022, FDA held a public meeting with its Pediatric Oncology Subcommittee of the Oncologic Drugs Advisory Committee to discuss the RACE Act, including challenges with same-in-class drugs.

Mary Denigan-Macauley Director, Health Care

Enclosure(s) – 2

Enclosure I: List of Molecular Targets and Associated Adult and Pediatric Indications in Planned Pediatric Studies

The FDA Reauthorization Act of 2017 includes a provision commonly known as the Research to Accelerate Cures and Equity for Children Act (RACE Act). The RACE Act requires sponsors of certain adult drugs that target cancer at the molecular level—referred to as molecularly targeted drugs—to submit plans to study the drug in the pediatric population (referred to as an initial pediatric study plan) to the Food and Drug Administration (FDA).[24] Included in these plans are the adult cancer that the adult drug is intended to treat, the associated molecular target—for example a protein present in a cancerous cell that is not present in a non-cancerous cell—and (when available) the pediatric cancer the sponsor plans to study. Table 2 provides this information for the five FDA-approved molecularly targeted adult cancer drugs since the implementation of the RACE Act (August 18, 2020) through August 18, 2022 with planned pediatric studies.

Enclosure II: Pediatric Study Requirement Waiver, Partial Waiver, and Deferral Justifications

The FDA Reauthorization Act of 2017 includes a provision commonly known as the Research to Accelerate Cures and Equity for Children Act (RACE Act).

[24] Pub. L. No. 115-52, § 504, 131 Stat. 1005, 1039-46 (codified in relevant part at 21 U.S.C. § 355c(e)). A sponsor means a person who takes responsibility for and initiates a clinical investigation. The sponsor may be an individual or pharmaceutical company, governmental agency, academic institution, private organization, or other organization. For the purposes of this report, we refer to both drugs and biologics as drugs. A molecularly targeted drug binds or interacts with the molecular target, thereby slowing or stopping the progression of cancer cell growth. For example, a drug may interact with a protein that is present in a cancerous cell but not present in a non-cancerous cell.

The RACE Act requires sponsors of certain adult drugs that target cancer at the molecular level—referred to as molecularly targeted drugs—to submit plans to study the drug in the pediatric population (referred to as an initial pediatric study plan) to the Food and Drug Administration (FDA) for review and agreement.[25] Sponsors are required to submit their initial pediatric study plan to FDA for review no later than 60 calendar days after the date of the end-of-phase 2 meeting, or at another time as agreed upon between FDA and the sponsor.[26]

Table 2. Cancer types and associated molecular targets for approved adult cancer drugs, August 18, 2020 through August 18, 2022

Pediatric cancer	Adult cancer	Molecular target[a]
Relapsed/refractory B-cell non-Hodgkin lymphoma	Relapsed/refractory diffuse large B- cell lymphoma	CD19
Recurrent/refractory low-grade glioma, other advanced solid tumors	Cholangiocarcinoma	FGFR
Relapsed/refractory tissue factor expressing tumors	Cervical cancer	F3 (Tissue Factor)
Melanoma	Melanoma	LAG3
Philadelphia chromosome positive chronic myeloid leukemia in chronic phase	Philadelphia chromosome positive chronic myeloid leukemia chronic phase	ABL1, ABL2

Source: GAO analysis of data provided by the Food and Drug Administration. | GAO-23-105947.

[a] A molecular target is a molecule involved in the growth or spread of cancer cells. A molecularly targeted drug binds or interacts with the molecular target, thereby slowing or stopping the progression of cancer cell growth. For example, a drug may interact with a protein that is present in a cancerous cell but not present in a non-cancerous cell.

---

[25] Pub. L. No. 115-52, § 504, 131 Stat. 1005, 1039-46 (codified in relevant part at 21 U.S.C. § 355c(e)). A sponsor means a person who takes responsibility for and initiates a clinical investigation. The sponsor may be an individual or pharmaceutical company, governmental agency, academic institution, private organization, or other organization. For the purposes of this report, we refer to both drugs and biologics as drugs. A molecularly targeted drug binds or interacts with the molecular target, thereby slowing or stopping the progression of cancer cell growth. For example, a drug may interact with a protein that is present in a cancerous cell but not present in a non-cancerous cell.

[26] The purpose of the end-of-phase 2 meetings is to determine the safety of proceeding to phase 3 clinical trials, to evaluate the phase 3 plan and protocols and the adequacy of current studies and plans to assess pediatric safety and effectiveness, and to identify any additional information necessary to support a marketing application for the uses under investigation.

In their initial pediatric study plans, sponsors may include a plan to request a full waiver, partial waiver, or deferral of pediatric study requirements.

- A full waiver means the sponsor does not need to conduct a pediatric study.
- A partial waiver allows the sponsor to exclude certain pediatric populations from the pediatric study. For example, if a drug is intended for patients who have failed existing treatment options, a sponsor may justify a planned request for a partial waiver for children under 1 year of age because they are unlikely to have exhausted available treatment options.
- A deferral allows sponsors with required pediatric studies to submit the study reports after the drug is approved for use in adults. Partial waivers and deferrals are not mutually exclusive—sponsors may receive a partial waiver and a deferral, allowing them to submit the reports for the pediatric study after the drug is approved for use in adults.[27]

Since the RACE Act was implemented on August 18, 2020 through August 18, 2022, there have been 53 initial pediatric study plans submitted to FDA for which FDA and the sponsor have agreed with the sponsor's plan to request a full waiver—meaning that a pediatric study would not have to be conducted.[28] See table 3 for the justifications for these full waivers.

---

[27] FDA reviews requests for full waivers, partial waivers, and deferrals in the initial pediatric study plan and makes a recommendation as to whether the requests meet statutory criteria when it agrees to the plan. FDA does not finalize its decision on any request for a waiver or deferral until it approves the drug for use in adults.

[28] According to data provided by FDA, of the 53 initial pediatric study plans for which FDA and the sponsor ultimately agreed with the sponsor's plan to request a full waiver, two did not initially include such a request. One sponsor initially requested a partial waiver but ultimately requested a full waiver, because the drug was a later generation product. Another sponsor initially requested a deferral but ultimately requested a full waiver, as the drug was deemed likely not to provide a meaningful therapeutic benefit over existing therapies for pediatric patients.

Table 3. Number of initial pediatric study plans with plans to request full waivers, and a justification, august 18, 2020 through August 18, 2022

Waiver justification	Number of initial pediatric study plans
Does not represent a meaningful therapeutic benefit over existing therapies for pediatric patients and is not likely to be used in a substantial number of pediatric patientsa	23
Evidence strongly suggests that the drug would be ineffective or unsafe in all pediatric age groups	1
Necessary studies are impossible or highly impracticable because, for example, the number of patients is so small or the patients are geographically dispersed	29
Total	53

Source: GAO analysis of data provided by the Food and Drug Administration (FDA). | GAO-23-105947.

Note: An initial pediatric study plan is a document that outlines the planned approach to study a drug in a pediatric population, which may include a plan to request a full waiver. A full waiver means the sponsor does not need to conduct a pediatric study. FDA reviews requests for full waivers in the initial pediatric study plan and makes a recommendation as to whether the request meets statutory criteria when it agrees to the plan. FDA does not finalize its decision on any request for a waiver until it approves the drug for use in adults.

[a] This category may also include some same-in-class drugs. According to FDA officials, same-in-class drugs are drugs that have the same molecular target and are in the same pharmacologic class, meaning they function similarly to each other.

During this same time period, sponsors have submitted 32 initial pediatric study plans to FDA for which FDA and the sponsor have agreed that a pediatric study will be conducted. However, 25 of these 32 include plans to request a partial waiver.[29] (See table 4.)

---

[29] According to data provided by FDA, of the 32 initial pediatric study plans, four of them originally included plans to request a full waiver. In these instances, FDA and the sponsor ultimately agreed that the sponsor would request a partial waiver (three drugs) or no waiver (one drug).

Table 4. Number of Initial Pediatric Study Plans with and without Plans to Request Partial Associated Justifications, August 18, Waive 2020 through August 18, 2022

Waiver type	Waiver justification	Number of initial pediatric study plans
	Does not represent a meaningful therapeutic benefit over existing therapies for pediatric patients in a specific pediatric age group and is not likely to be used by a substantial number of pediatric patients in that age group.	1
Partial waiver	Necessary studies are impossible or highly impracticable in a specific pediatric age group, such as infants.	21
	There is evidence strongly suggesting that the drug would be ineffective or unsafe in a specific pediatric age group.	3
Subtotal (partial waiver)		25
No waiver	Not applicable	7
Total (partial waiver and no wavier)		32

Source: GAO analysis of data provided by the Food and Drug Administration (FDA). | GAO-23-105947.

Note: An initial pediatric study plan is a document that outlines the planned approach to study a drug in a pediatric population, which may include a plan to request a partial waiver. A partial waiver means that the sponsor is not required to conduct a pediatric study for some pediatric patients. For example, a partial waiver may result in a sponsor not studying the drug in pediatric patients under the age of one. FDA reviews requests for partial waivers in the initial pediatric study plan and makes a recommendation as to whether the request meets statutory criteria when it agrees to the plan. FDA does not finalize its decision on any request for a waiver until it approves the drug for use in adults.

Further, of the 32 initial pediatric study plans, 30 include plans to request a deferral.[30] (Some sponsors may request a partial waiver and a deferral.) See table 5 for the justification of these deferrals.

Table 5. Number of initial pediatric study plans with plans to request defer justifications, August 18, 2020 through August 18, 2022

Deferral justification	Number of initial pediatric study plans
Pediatric studies should be delayed until additional safety or effectiveness data have been collected	14
Drug is ready for approval for use in adults before the pediatric study is completed	16
Total	30

Source: GAO analysis of data provided by the Food and Drug Administration (FDA). | GAO-23-105947.

Note: An initial pediatric study plan is a document that outlines the planned approach to study a drug in a pediatric population, which may include a plan to request a deferral. A deferral allows sponsors with planned pediatric studies to submit the study reports after the drug is approved for adults. FDA reviews requests for deferrals in the initial pediatric study plan and makes a recommendation as to whether the request meets statutory criteria when it agrees to the plan. FDA does not finalize its decision on any request for a deferral until it approves the drug for use in adults.

30 According to data provided by FDA, 27 sponsors initially requested deferrals in their pediatric study plans. Of those 27, FDA agreed with 26 sponsors' plans to request a deferral. In one instance, FDA and the sponsor ultimately agreed that the sponsor would request a full waiver. Additionally, there were four sponsors that initially requested full waivers, but ultimately agreed with FDA to request deferred studies—three sponsors ultimately requested planned partial waivers and deferrals, and one ultimately requested a planned deferral.

Chapter 12

Declines in Cancer Death Rates Among Youth: United States, 2001–2021*

Sally C. Curtin
and Robert N. Anderson

Keywords: malignant neoplasms, death certificates, underlying cause of death, National Vital Statistics System

Key Findings

Data from the National Vital Statistics System

- From 2001 to 2021, the cancer death rate for youth ages 0–19 years in the United States declined 24%, from 2.75 to 2.10 per 100,000.
- Declines between 2001 and 2011 in cancer death rates occurred for all age groups (0–4, 5–9, 10–14, and 15–19 years), but only rates among those ages 0–4 and 5–9 declined through 2021.
- Declines between 2001 and 2011 in cancer death rates occurred for Black non-Hispanic, White non-Hispanic (subsequently, White), and Hispanic youth, but only rates for White youth continued to decline through 2021.

---

* This is an edited, reformatted and augmented version of Data Brief of U.S. Department of Health & Human Services, Centers for Disease Control and Prevention, National Center for Health Statistics, Publication No. No. 484, dated November 2023.

In: Understanding Cancer
Editor: Angela C. Ray
ISBN: 979-8-89530-769-4

- Brain cancer was the most common cancer causing death in youth in 2021, with a rate (0.59) that was 23% higher than the rate for leukemia (0.48) and more than twice that of bone and articular cartilage cancer (0.25).

Since the mid-1970s, cancer death rates for youth in the United States have declined significantly despite a slow increase in incidence for some of the major types (1–3). A previous report with trends from 1999 through 2014 showed declines for all 5-year age groups of youth (0–4, 5–9, 10–14, 15–19) (4). This Data Brief updates that report by presenting trends in cancer death rates through 2021. Rates from 2001 to 2021 are presented in total and for females and males. Rates for 2001, 2011, and 2021 are presented by 5-year age groups and for White, Black, and Hispanic youth. Trends are shown for the three most common types of cancer in youth.

Between 2001 and 2021, Cancer Death Rates Declined for Both Female and Male Youth Ages 0–19 Years

- The cancer death rate for youth ages 0–19 years was 24% lower in 2021 (2.10 per 100,000) than in 2001 (2.75) (Figure 1).
- Cancer death rates declined for both female and male youth between 2001 and 2021, by 30% for females (from 2.50 to 1.76) and 19% for males (from 2.99 to 2.42).
- From 2020 to 2021, the cancer death rate for male youth increased 8% (from 2.25 to 2.42), while the rate for females declined 9% (from 1.94 to 1.76).
- During 2001, 2011, and 2021, cancer death rates for male youth ranged from 20–38% higher than females, with the largest percentage difference in 2021.

Cancer Death Rates Declined Between 2001 And 2011 for All Age Groups of Youth

- Youth in all age groups (0–4, 5–9, 10–14, and 15–19) experienced declines in cancer death rates between 2001 and 2011, but only those ages 0–4 and 5–9 had significant declines between 2011 and 2021 (Figure 2).

- In 2001, 2011, and 2021, adolescents ages 15–19 had the highest cancer death rates of all age groups of youth, although the rate for this group was 23% lower in 2021 (2.75 per 100,000) than in 2001 (3.58).
- In 2001 and 2011, cancer death rates for youth ages 0–4, 5–9, and 10–14 were not significantly different; by 2021, the rate for adolescents ages 10–14 (2.09) was higher than for children ages 0–4 (1.77) and 5–9 (1.71).

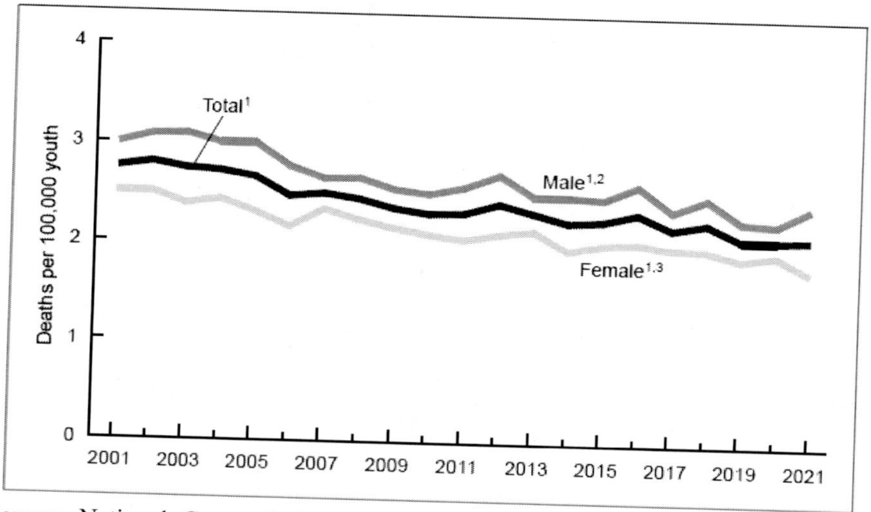

Source: National Center for Health Statistics, National Vital Statistics System, mortality data file.

Notes: Cancer deaths are identified with International Classification of Diseases, 10th Revision underlying cause-of-death codes C00–C97. Access data table for Figure 1 at: https://www.cdc.gov/nchs/data/databriefs/db484-tables.pdf#1.

[1]Significantly decreasing trend from 2001 to 2021 ($p < 0.05$).

[2]Rate in 2021 significantly higher than in 2020 ($p < 0.05$).

[3]Rate in 2021 significantly lower than in 2020 ($p < 0.05$).

Figure 1. Cancer death rate for youth ages 0–19 years, by sex: United States, 2001 to 2021.

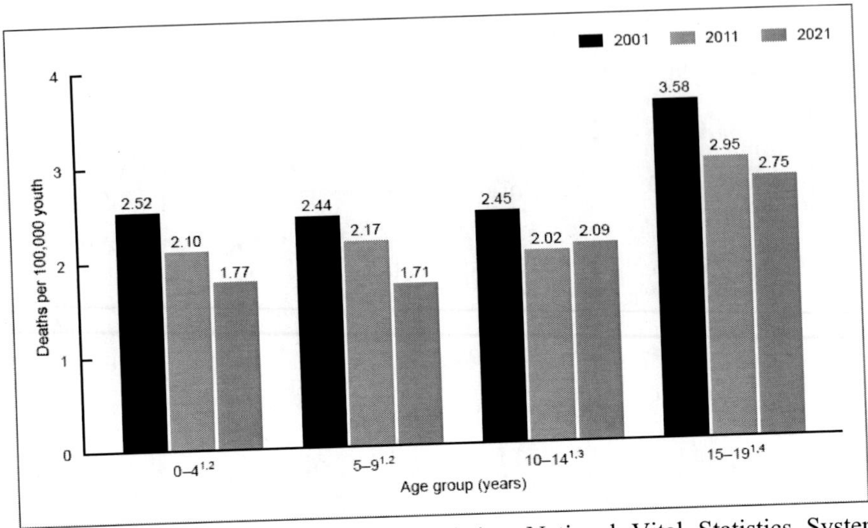

Source: National Center for Health Statistics, National Vital Statistics System, mortality data file.

Notes: Cancer deaths are identified with International Classification of Diseases, 10th Revision underlying cause-of-death codes C00–C97. Access data table for Figure 2 at: https://www.cdc.gov/nchs/data/databriefs/db484-tables.pdf#2.

[1] Rate in 2011 significantly lower than in 2001 ($p < 0.05$).

[2] Rate in 2021 significantly lower than in 2011 ($p < 0.05$).

[3] Rate in 2021 significantly higher than for 0–4 years and 5–9 ($p < 0.05$).

[4] Rates significantly higher than rate for other age groups ($p < 0.05$).

Figure 2. Cancer death rate for youth ages 0–19 years, by age group: United States, 2001, 2011, and 2021.

In 2021, The Cancer Death Rate for White Youth Was Lower Than for Black and Hispanic Youth

- Percentage declines between 2001 and 2011 in cancer death rates were similar among Black non-Hispanic (subsequently, Black), White non-Hispanic (subsequently, White), and Hispanic youth, ranging from 15 to 17% (Figure 3).
- The cancer death rate for White youth declined 12% from 2011 through 2021 (from 2.27 to 1.99 per 100,000), while rates for Black and Hispanic youth did not change significantly.
- In 2001 and 2011, differences in cancer death rates among Black, White, and Hispanic youth were not statistically significant. In 2021,

the rate for White youth was 15%–16% lower than for Black and Hispanic youth.

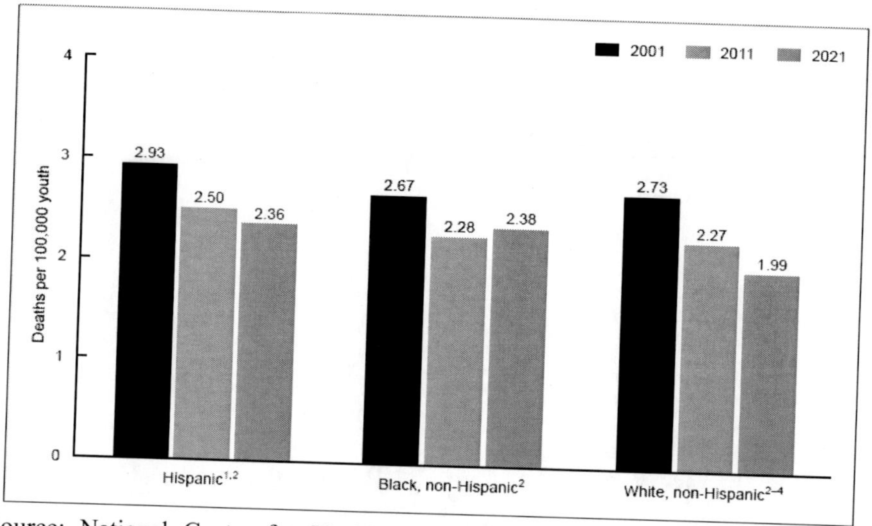

Source: National Center for Health Statistics, National Vital Statistics System, mortality data file.

Notes: Cancer deaths are identified with International Classification of Diseases, 10th Revision underlying cause-of-death codes C00–C97. Access data table for Figure 3 at: https://www.cdc.gov/nchs/data/databriefs/db484-tables.pdf#3.

[1] People of Hispanic origin may be of any race.

[2] Rate in 2011 significantly lower than in 2001 ($p < 0.05$).

[3] Rate in 2021 significantly lower than in 2011 ($p < 0.05$).

[4] Rate in 2021 significantly lower than for Black non-Hispanic and Hispanic ($p < 0.05$).

Figure 3. Cancer death rate for youth ages 0–19 years, by race and Hispanic origin: United States, 2001, 2011, and 2021.

In 2021, Brain Cancer Was the Most Common Type of Cancer Causing Death in Youth

- Death rates among youth due to leukemia, the most common type of cancer causing death in youth in 2001, declined 47% between 2001 and 2021, from 0.90 per 100,000 to 0.48 (Figure 4).
- Brain cancer death rates did not change significantly between 2001 and 2011 but declined by 11% from 2011 (0.65) to 2021 (0.59).

- Among youth, cancer death rates due to bone and articular cartilage cancer declined from
- 0.23 to 0.21 during 2001–2011 but then increased to 0.25 through 2021.
- Brain cancer was the leading type of cancer causing death in youth in 2021, with a death rate that was 23% higher than for leukemia and more than twice that of bone and articular cancer.

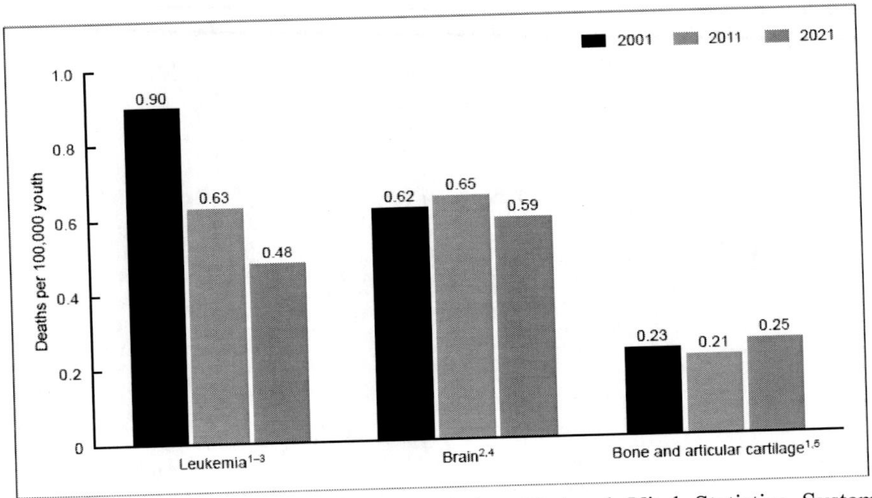

Source: National Center for Health Statistics, National Vital Statistics System, mortality data file.

Notes: Cancer deaths are identified with International Classification of Diseases, 10th Revision underlying cause-of-death codes leukemia (C91–C95), brain (C71), and bone and articular cartilage (C40–C41). Access data table for Figure 4 at: https://www.cdc.gov/nchs/data/databriefs/db484-tables.pdf#4.

[1] Rate in 2011 significantly lower than in 2001 ($p < 0.05$).

[2] Rate in 2021 significantly lower than in 2011 ($p < 0.05$).

[3] Rate in 2001 significantly higher than for all other groups ($p < 0.05$). 4Rate in 2021 significantly higher than for all other groups ($p < 0.05$). 5Rate in 2021 significantly higher than in 2011 ($p < 0.05$).

Figure 4. Cancer death rate for youth ages 0–19 years, by the three most common types of cancer in youth: United States, 2001, 2011, and 2021.

Summary

Cancer mortality in youth continued to decline during 2001–2021, building on progress of the previous 3 decades (1–4). The overall cancer death rate declined by one-fourth during 2001–2021, with a greater percentage decline for females (30%) than males (19%). All 5-year age groups experienced declines from 2001 to 2011, but only the younger age groups (0–4 and 5–9 years) experienced significant declines from 2011 to 2021. White, Black, and Hispanic youth had similar cancer death rates in 2001 and 2011. However, the rate for White youth continued to decline from 2011 to 2021, while rates for Black and Hispanic youth remained stable. As such, in 2021, the rate for White youth was significantly lower than for Black and Hispanic youth. Leukemia had been the most common type of cancer causing death in youth in 2001 but declined by 47% over the period. Despite an 11% decline in the second half of the period, brain cancer was the leading type of cancer causing death in youth in 2021. Death rates due to bone and articular cancer increased from 2011 to 2021.

Data Source and Methods

Mortality and population data are from the National Center for Health Statistics 1999–2020 underlying cause-of-death bridged-race files and 2018–2021 underlying cause-of-death single-race files (5). Population data for 2001–2009 are based on July 1 intercensal estimates, and for 2011–2020 they are July 1 postcensal estimates based on the 2020 census. Population estimates for 2021 are estimated as of July 1 based on the Blended Base produced by the U.S.

Census Bureau in lieu of the April 1, 2020, decennial population count. The Blended Base is a blend of vintage 2020 postcensal population estimates, 2020 Demographic Analysis estimates, and the 2020 Census PL 94-171 Redistricting File (6). Cancer deaths are those with International Classification of Diseases, 10th Revision underlying cause-of-death codes C00–C97 (7). Cancer deaths by specific anatomical site are classified as follows: leukemia (C91–C95), brain cancer (C71), and bone and articular cartilage (C40–C41).

Trends in Figure 1 were evaluated using the Joinpoint Regression Program (8). The Joinpoint software was used to fit weighted least-squares regression models to the estimated proportions on the logarithmic scale. The default settings allowed for as few as three observed time points in the beginning, ending, and middle line segments, including the joinpoints. Using these settings, a maximum of three joinpoints were searched for using the grid search algorithm and permutation test, using an overall alpha level of 0.05. Pairwise comparisons of rates shown in Figures 2–4 were tested using the test statistic at $p < 0.05$.

This report features data for the three largest race and ethnicity groups (White, Black, and Hispanic), which comprised 92% of all cancer deaths in youth in 2021. Data are not shown for American Indian and Alaska Native non-Hispanic, Asian non-Hispanic, and Native Hawaiian and Other Pacific Islander non-Hispanic people due to small sample sizes in some years that can result in unreliable rates. Information on race and ethnicity are from death certificates and are supplied by an informant, usually the next of kin. Race and Hispanic origin are two distinct attributes and are reported separately on death certificates. As such, the data shown in this report by Hispanic origin and race are based on a combination of the two attributes for the non-Hispanic population. Data shown for the Hispanic population include youth of any race. Death rates for Hispanic people are impacted by inconsistencies in reporting Hispanic origin on the death certificate compared with censuses and surveys. A validity study has shown underreporting on death certificates of Hispanic decedents by 3% (9). However, this underreporting was not found for Hispanic decedents under age 25. Rates in this report for 2001 and 2011 are based on multiple-race mortality data that were bridged to single-race categories based on the 1977 Office of Management and Budget standards for the classification of race and ethnicity. Rates for 2021 were based on the 1997 Office of Management and Budget standards and might differ slightly compared with the 1977 standards (10).

About the Authors

Sally C. Curtin and Robert N. Anderson are with the National Center for Health Statistics, Division of Vital Statistics.

References

[1] Siegel R. L., Miller K. D., Wagle N. S., Jemal A. Cancer statistics, 2023. *Ca Cancer J.* 73:17–48. 2023.

[2] Ries L. A. G., Smith M. A., Gurney J. G., Linet M, Tamra T., Young J. L., Bunin G. R. Cancer incidence and survival among children and adolescents: United States SEER program 1975–1995, *National Cancer Institute, SEER program.* NIH Pub. No. 99-4649. 1999.

[3] Cronin K. A., Scott S., Firth A. U., Sung H., Henley J. S., Sherman R. L., et al. Annual report to the nation on the status of cancer, part 1: National cancer statistics. *Cancer* 128(24):4251–84. 2022.

[4] Curtin S. C., Miniño A. M., Anderson R. N. Declines in cancer death rates among children and adolescents in the United States, 1999–2014. NCHS Data Brief, no 257. Hyattsville, *MD: National Center for Health Statistics.* 2016. Available from: https://www.cdc.gov/nchs/products/ databriefs/ db257.htm.

[5] National Center for Health Statistics. CDC WONDER. 1999–2020 underlying cause of death by bridged-race categories. 2018–2021 underlying cause of death by single-race categories. 2023. Available from: https://wonder.cdc.gov/Deaths-by-Underlying-Cause.html.

[6] U.S. Census Bureau. Methodology for the United States population estimates: vintage 2021 nation, states, counties, and Puerto Rico–April 1, 2020 to July 1, 2021. 2021. Available from: https://www2.census.gov/programs-surveys/popest/technical-documentation/methodology/2020-2021/methods-statement-v2021.pdf.

[7] World Health Organization. International statistical classification of diseases and related health problems, 10th revision (ICD–10). 2008 ed. 2009.

[8] National Cancer Institute. Joinpoint Regression Program (Version 4.9.0.0) [computer software]. 2021.

[9] Arias E, Heron M, Hakes JK. The validity of race and Hispanic-origin reporting on death certificates in the United States: An update. National Center for Health Statistics. Vital Health Stat 2(172). 2016. Available from: https://www.cdc.gov/nchs/data/series/sr_02/sr02_172.pdf.

[10] Heron M. Comparability of race-specific mortality data based on 1977 versus 1997 reporting standards. National Vital Statistics Reports; vol 70 no 3. Hyattsville, MD: National Center for Health Statistics. 2021. Available from: https://www.cdc.gov/nchs/data/nvsr/nvsr70/nvsr70-03-508.pdf.

Suggested Citation

Curtin SC, Anderson RN. Declines in cancer death rates among youth: United States, 2001–2021.

NCHS Data Brief, no 484. Hyattsville, MD: National Center for Health Statistics. 2023. DOI: https://dx.doi.org/10.15620/cdc:134499.

Copyright Information

National Center for Health Statistics

Brian C. Moyer, Ph.D., Director
Amy M. Branum, Ph.D., Associate Director for Science

Division of Vital Statistics

Paul D. Sutton, Ph.D.,
Acting Director

Andrés A. Berruti, Ph.D., M.A.,
Associate Director for Science

Index

A

B

C

D

E

F

G

Q

R

S